Bodyfulness

Bodyfulness

Somatic Practices for
Presence, Empowerment, and
Waking Up in This Life

CHRISTINE CALDWELL, PhD

Foreword by David I. Rome

SHAMBHALA
Boulder
2018

Shambhala Publications, Inc.
2129 13th Street
Boulder, Colorado 80302
www.shambhala.com

Small portions of the introduction, chapter 1, and chapter 7 were adapted from Christine Caldwell, "Mindfulness and Bodyfulness: A New Paradigm," *Journal of Contemplative Inquiry* 1, no. 1 (2014): 77–96. Small portions of chapter 5 were adapted from Himmat Kaur Victoria and Christine Caldwell, "Breathwork in Body Psychotherapy: Towards a More Unified Theory and Practice," *Body, Movement and Dance in Psychotherapy* 6, no. 2 (2011): 89–101. Small portions of chapter 8 were adapted from chapter 2 of *Oppression and the Body: Roots, Resistances, and Reclamations,* ed. Christine Caldwell and Lucia Bennett Leighton (Berkeley: North Atlantic Books, 2018): 31–50.

9 8 7 6 5 4 3

Printed in the United States of America

Shambhala Publications makes every effort to print on acid-free, recycled paper.

Shambhala Publications is distributed worldwide by Penguin Random House, Inc., and its subsidiaries.

Designed by Claudine Mansour Design

LIBRARY OF CONGRESS CATALOGING-IN-PUBLICATION DATA
Names: Caldwell, Christine, 1952– author.
Title: Bodyfulness: somatic practices for presence, empowerment, and waking up in this life / Christine Caldwell.
Description: Boulder: Shambhala, 2018. | Includes bibliographical references and index.
Identifiers: LCCN 2018006101 | ISBN 9781611805109 (pbk.: alk. paper)
Subjects: LCSH: Mind and body therapies.
Classification: LCC RC489.M53 C34 2018 | DDC 616.89/1—dc23
LC record available at https://lccn.loc.gov/2018006101

For my grandson,
Cooper
And my daughter-in-law,
Brianna

Contents

Foreword

IT TAKES AUDACITY to coin a new word in the English language. Wouldn't *somatic awareness* or *embodied mindfulness* have sufficed to describe the territory Christine Caldwell illuminates in this book? Do we really need the neologism *bodyfulness*? At face value, bodyfulness presents itself as the opposite of mindfulness. However, Caldwell's intention here is subtler and more subversive. Because mind/body dualism has become so entrenched in our conceptual library, *mindfulness* as a term cannot avoid reaffirming the cultural bias that mind is superior to body. This is why we need a completely new term. *Bodyfulness* overcomes the bias toward the mental, while at the same time extending and greatly enriching the signification of mindfulness itself.

In fact, Christine Caldwell's approach is extraordinary in the breadth of its concerns. Her knowledge of the field itself is comprehensive—the Additional Notes and References section alone is a tour de force—and she enlarges its relevance to today's society through her passionate embrace of the themes of contemplative awareness, ethical action, and social equity.

Bodyfulness begins when the embodied self is held in a conscious, contemplative environment. It's then coupled with nonjudgmental engagement with bodily processes, an acceptance and appreciation of one's bodily nature, and an ethical and aesthetic orientation toward taking right actions physically so that a lessening of suffering and an increase in human and nonhuman potential may emerge.

That is probably the most nuanced of several definitions of bodyfulness Caldwell offers. At another point she describes it more experientially:

The body isn't a thing we have but an experience we are. Bodyfulness is about working toward our potential as a whole human animal that breathes as well as thinks, moves as well as sits still, takes action as well as considers, and exists not just because it thinks but because it dances, stretches, bounces, gazes, focuses, and attunes to others.

Elsewhere she captures the essence of bodyfulness, memorably, in three words: "attention during action."

The book begins by articulating eight core principles of body processes. The first, oscillation, provides a key to the other seven—and indeed to the whole book. The living body and its interdependent systems like respiration, digestion, circulation, and the nervous system are in a continual movement, without which the body cannot maintain its equilibrium. The heart contracts and releases, contracts and releases; the rate at which it does so speeds up and slows down in response to how much work the body has to do. Each physiological system oscillates along its own continuum of activity, and all of them oscillate interdependently, like the different instruments in an orchestra modulating between loud and soft, fast and slow, high and low notes, each following its own part in the score yet all together making an intricate, coherent, harmonious whole.

The body as a whole is a continuum of processes that range from those that are completely unconscious to those that we are fully conscious and in control of. As Caldwell demonstrates both in her topic-by-topic presentations and in their accompanying exercises, it is in the middle of this range, where previously unconscious functions and longstanding habitual patterns can be brought into the light of awareness, that somatic practices are particularly powerful. It is here too that Caldwell articulates what is probably her most original and important contribution to the field of somatic psychology: the vital role of embodied contemplative awareness.

Bodyfulness involves a purposeful and athletic ability to alter our attentional focus so that the amount and type of sensations we work with can be nourishing and deeply informative . . . While thinking evokes the mind, moving evokes the body. Movement and action form the system through which the body knows, identifies, remembers, and contemplates itself.

The second part of the book lays out four essential body functions—sensing, breathing, moving, and relating—together with a menu of exercises for each. The instructions for these exercises are easy to follow, thorough, and precise, and at the same time suffused with contemplative and experiential wisdom. Here is how Caldwell concludes her description of the Balanced Breath practice:

It's important not to force [the pause at the end of the out-breath] to happen, as this defeats the physiological pause and disrupts the relaxation of the cycle. Simply watch for and greet

the pause if it shows up, and bear witness as your body organizes itself to inhale again on its own physiological authority . . .
[N]otice what associations emerge . . . as any conscious breathing
will bring up potentially powerful and useful contemplations.

Caldwell differentiates bodyfulness from *embodiment*, an important word that, like mindfulness, has become rusty through
overuse:

In embodiment we know what we feel and sense, but in bodyfulness we somatically reflect upon and even challenge our
embodied experience in a way that tempers our compelling and
habituated action patterns as well as our experiments with abusing power.

It is here Caldwell challenges the mind's superiority over the body
as an article of faith common to "civilized" societies. It is part and
parcel of the self-serving and toxic belief that "man" holds heavenly
sanctioned "dominion" over the animals (let alone plants and fun-
gi). While the human capacity for cognition and metacognition is
undoubtedly a supreme evolutionary achievement (for better and
for worse, it becomes increasingly evident), the roots and purposes
of human cognition lie entirely with the physical body. Mind is an
outgrowth of and in service to the same life process that we share
with all living organisms.

In overturning millennia of "mindism," Caldwell not only creates new terms, she also resituates old ones:

Awareness will not be categorized as a function of mind but as
a function of sensory and motoric processing, so that sensory

awareness becomes one of our greatest allies in the work of moving toward bodyful states.

She works a similar reorientation in the meaning of *emotional intelligence*, a coinage given wide currency by Daniel Goleman's hugely influential 1995 book of that title:

> Our emotional intelligence, however, is mostly measured by how in touch we are with our feeling, moving, and communicating body. When we want to know how we *really feel*, we typically need to check in with what we are *really doing*—our breathing pace and pattern, the tension in our face, the tone of our voice, the flutters in our stomach.

And about physical fitness—the signature obsession of the bicycling, yoga, and Pilates mecca that is Boulder, Colorado, where Caldwell has spent the last thirty-five years teaching at Naropa University—she pointedly says, "Pedaling on an exercise bike while checking our emails likely generates some benefit, but it's not cultivating bodyfulness."

In the book's third and final part, "Bodyful Applications and Actions," Caldwell foregrounds the social critique and activist thrust that percolate through the previous parts. She engages the more socially oriented issues of body identity, body authority, and bodily-sourced activism. And in her most acute critique of contemporary culture, she describes the opposite of bodyfulness, *bodylessness*, which is characterized by:

> ... four conditions: (1) ignoring the body, (2) seeing the body as an object or project, (3) hating the body, and (4) making one's

own or other people's bodies wrong. The result of bodylessness is a life lived at a distance from who we were, who we are, and who we will be. This distance from ourselves causes us to suffer more, feel less pleasure, treat others poorly, and experience more challenges in living a self-reflective life.

Lest her activist intentions be missed, Caldwell tells us that "using the word *bodyful* may be as much a political act as a literary or poetic device." In pursuit of this sociopolitical mission, she is also realigning our understanding of contemplative practice. In an age when civilization itself seems to have lost its way, contemplation cannot hold itself apart from an ethical imperative to work for societal change. UN Secretary General Dag Hammarskjöld, a deeply contemplative man who sacrificed his life in pursuit of peace and justice for the world, said: "In our age, the road to holiness necessarily passes through the world of action." In the final chapter, "The Enlightened Body," Caldwell echoes and amplifies Hammarskjöld's precept:

While sitting on a cushion or kneeling in prayer brings with it many health benefits and contemplative insights, how we get up off the cushion, floor, or pew and navigate our daily life requires the breathing, moving, sensing, and relating body. Reflection without action doesn't change anything because the feedback loop of contemplative inner experience and contemplative outer action demands that we stay the course, that we stay with the sequence such that our body literally enacts its awakened state. Only then is enlightenment truly a light in the world, one that shines both inward and outward.

Over the past fifty years, the field of somatic psychology, or body psychotherapy, has grown from modest and disparate beginnings into a rich and multifaceted body of theory and methodology. *Bodyfulness* is a groundbreaking guide to principles and practices of somatic healing and personal empowerment presented by one of the field's leading academic and clinical practitioners. It is at once a hands-on manual suitable for beginners, a rich resource for somatically-oriented trainers and counselors, and a heartfelt call for humanity to wake up to the untapped resources our bodies hold for living more fulfilling, wise, and ethical lives. I fell in love with this book, and when in love one wants to linger. Whether you are after the hands-on, self-help utility *Bodyfulness* offers or want to delve into the deeper theoretical ideas Caldwell provides, this book is one you may well fall in love with too.

> —DAVID I. ROME, author of *Your Body Knows the Answer: Using Your Felt Sense to Solve Problems, Effect Change, and Liberate Creativity*

Acknowledgments

THIS BOOK IS itself like a body, a body that has been nourished and cared for by many other bodies. In the tradition of my teacher Thich Nhat Hanh, I would like to bow in deep gratitude to my parents, Jim and Lucille Caldwell, who gave me life, home, values, and integrity.

I don't think I could understand *bodyfulness* in any substantive way without the love, support, and friendship of my family: my husband, Jack Haggerty; my sister, Ann; my brother Jim; my brother-in-law, Gary and sister-in-law, Jan; my son, Jesse Caldwell Silver; my incredible daughter-in-law, Brianna Silver; and my magnificent grandson, Cooper Caldwell Silver.

Deep bows go to my teachers, Sophie Darbonne, Allen Darbonne, Allegra Fuller Snyder, Alma Hawkins, Judith Aston, and Thich Nhat Hanh.

I place my hands together to honor Naropa University. Thank you for sheltering and nurturing and challenging me for over thirty-five years. And many thanks to my editor, Kathleen Gregory, for her patience, insight, and generosity.

I bow at last to my friends and colleagues, too numerous to mention. To try anyway, I want to express profound gratitude to Naropa's Somatic Counseling Leadership Team: Wendy Allen, Mike Lythgoe, Carla Sherrell, Himmat K. Victoria, Ryan Kennedy, Zoe Avestreih, and Deb Silver. They create a true holding environment for creativity, intellect, play, emotional regulation, and best of all, bodyful living.

My dear friend Ursa Spaete Schumacher carefully read the entire manuscript and gave me thoughtful and caring feedback, much of which was immediately incorporated into the book. Thank you, thank you, thank you!

I'm very grateful for the shelter and atmosphere of the Boulder Public Library, within whose walls much of this book was written. And riding my bike six miles one way to the library put me in a great mood for writing about the body, along with all those NIA dance classes.

Many friends and colleagues have stood up for me and for this book. Thank you so much to Marc Bekoff, Rae Johnson, Carly Parry, Pat Ogden, Ursa Spaete Schumacher, Ute Lang, Gretl Bauer, Barbara Schmidt Rohr, Thomas von Stuckrad, Elmar Kruithoff, Jayne Satter, Terrell, Malie, and Kekuni Minton, Melanie Smithson, the late Don Campbell, and to "the Hamburg Group." This is our body.

Introduction
Why Bodyfulness?

AN OLD WOMAN sits at a bus stop, and as she waits she scans the sky, noticing the gradations of color in the clouds. Beside her a child stands, bouncing up and down on his toes and noticing the muscles he is using to balance himself. Across town, a man sits in a meditation class, noticing the details of his breathing. In the next building, an office worker has a headache and is working with it by drinking more water, relaxing, and stretching her neck. Across the street, in a dance studio, a trio of dancers improvise different movements, attending both to their own movements as well as attuning to the movements of the other two, working to find ones that have aesthetic and symbolic significance. All these people are embedding themselves in their bodily experience, perhaps for just a moment, in passing, or perhaps as a dedicated practice. Their attention focuses on their senses and their actions, an awareness of both being and doing. Perhaps they are also being bodyful.

In English, the word *bodyfulness* strikes most of us as odd and awkward. Why is that, aside from the fact that it's not in the dictionary? How can I be "full" of body? The word *bodyfulness* has been bandied around for a while.[1] Other "fullness" words in the English language are in general use, such as *thoughtfulness*, *heartfulness*, and *soulfulness*. These "fullness" words connote positive human traits we all want to cultivate. They imply caring, consideration, sincerity, deep reflection, loving-kindness, and engagement with deeper places within oneself.

Humans invent words because we need language to articulate and share our experience with others, yet our words also actively shape how we perceive and move in the world. Most of our language is given to us by family, culture, and society, shaping our identity every time we use it by boxing up our thoughts, feelings, and experiences into predetermined categories. However, just like "the map is not the territory," our words are always maplike approximations of our bodily experiences. They will sooner or later fail us in the face of our vast and wordlessly articulate lived experiences. Yet it's the wordless body that makes our words meaningful.

These word maps can be redrawn in response to our ongoing experiences: during meditation or therapy, while experiencing art, or as a result of a traumatic experience. These moments can be disorienting, as they can rattle and potentially reshuffle our internal dictionaries and our very identities. Part of leading a self-reflective life involves reflecting on the words we use to express ourselves and making sure they still describe our direct experiences and the world around us as best they can.

This book turns to the wordless and ineffable body as a means of guiding us along that path of lexical and experiential reflection, because it's the body that makes this contemplative process so effective. Within the lived experience of our body we can feel and express directly, creating a powerful and direct locating of ourselves in the present moment. This is bodyfulness.

Bodyfulness and the more popular term *mindfulness* are related to each other. The word *mindfulness* is a recent translation from the ancient Pali language, and incorporates states of awareness, attention, and remembering. It's only in the last twenty or so years that both the term and the practice of mindfulness have taken hold in popular Western culture. An unintended result of this helpful development, however, has been the popularization of a somewhat ill-defined and overgeneralized term. It was shaking out a more accurate meaning of *mindfulness* that got this book started.

Contemporary understandings of mindfulness describe it most simply as "moment-by-moment awareness." Yet we tend to assume this process involves a mind being aware of both its own thoughts and its body. When we use this word in this way, it's hard not to categorize the mind as related to thoughts and inner words, as rationality and logic. The word *contemplate*, for instance, typically means to think about or to be thoughtful. Though we often profess that an awakened and self-reflective life involves much more than thoughtfulness, here in the West we tend to centralize and valorize the mind when we use the word *mindfulness*. Because of this tendency, mindfulness is in danger of marginalizing our bodily experiences and perpetuating a false dualism between our physical and cognitive selves.

Eastern traditions typically don't separate the mind from the body but treat mind-body unity as an achievement rather than an essential state. This unity must be physically as well as intellectually cultivated. The Japanese philosopher Yuasa Yasuo, for instance, felt that knowledge can only occur through bodily recognition or realization, and he believed that this realization occurs only after engaging in body practices (such as tai chi, yoga, and the like) alongside meditation. He defined mind-body unity as the minimal distance between the movement of the mind and the movement of the body.[2]

Here in the West we don't have a distinct word to express this cultivated unity, nor one that expresses a state of being fully physical

—a deep state of somatic wakefulness, of profound occupation of the present moment as it manifests in flesh, nerve, and bone. More recently in the West, philosophers, scientists, and psychotherapists have been working on this issue by using terms such as *heightened somatic awareness, body sense, somaesthetics, embodied and enactive cognition, wordlessly shared intersubjective relating and knowing*, and the *body-to-body transmission of healing*, to name a few (see the notes section at the end of the book for more details).

The word *bodyfulness* shakes up these discourses. It questions the idea that the mind and body are unified or cultivated. It asserts that we *are* a body and that the mind is one of the many activities that human evolution creates, just as it creates heartbeats, brain waves, and breath. Western philosophy toyed with a similar idea, mostly in the nineteenth century, calling it *materialism*[3] In materialism we are a thing, an object much like a machine, no more and no less. This extreme position helped push back against the excesses of superstition and spiritual/religious abuse that ran rampant during previous centuries. Yet leaving no room for the mysterious, the transcendent, and the realities of consciousness carries its own excesses.

While this book works with the idea that we are all and simply bodies, what a body *is* can be seen quite differently. Our body isn't a machine. Life has imbued it with faculties that allow it to contemplate itself and to extend itself, to the point where we now are increasingly taking charge of our body's own evolution. We are awakening our bodies—ourselves—in evermore meaningful ways. As a contemplative practice, bodyfulness literally and metaphorically can provide us with the principles that will help us keep waking up.

I'm using the word *bodyfulness* so that we can celebrate our diverse, awakening bodies within social contexts as well as our own interior landscapes, locations the body has long deserved to occupy but hasn't achieved in most modern cultures, especially Western ones. Perhaps this is because bodyfulness has been so ineffable that we just didn't want to box it up until now. But more likely it's because we can't name something that we don't regularly know how to feel, that isn't important to us, or that we actively marginalize.

This book is about inventing a new word so that something important might be valued and communicated among us. It's about inventing a new word so that certain valuable experiences and states can become more coherent, supported, and accessible to more people on a daily basis. It's about finding a more accurate home for body-based contemplative practices. It's about foregrounding an unrealized aspect of human potential that just might have a profound effect on our future.

The Contemplative Body

Bodyfulness is at its heart a contemplative practice, and this distinguishes it from embodiment. *Embodiment* is the closest term to *bodyfulness* that we have had up until now. The word *embodiment* refers to our ability to rest our care and attention into our direct, immediate experience on a consistent basis. Bodyfulness, however, is more than just embodiment. I would define embodiment as awareness of and attentive participation with the body's states and actions. Bodyfulness begins when the embodied self is held in a conscious, contemplative environment. It's then coupled with nonjudgmental engagement with bodily processes, an acceptance and appreciation of one's bodily nature, and an ethical and aesthetic orientation toward taking right actions physically so that a lessening of suffering and an increase in human and nonhuman potential may emerge. This attentive engagement cultivates bodyfulness over time. Just as the psychologist Abraham Maslow noted that all humans, when they reach a threshold of safety, security, and belonging, endeavor to fully realize their potential, so embodiment can be seen as a basic human need and right that can occur naturally. Bodyfulness can come to represent our disciplined efforts to more fully self-realize our physical nature. How then do we physically self-realize?

We move. While thinking evokes the mind, moving evokes the body. Movement and action form the system through which the body knows, identifies, remembers, and contemplates itself, and it's this somewhat ineffable territory that this book will explore. We are bodies that are always moving. The practice of moving while being aware, moment by moment, is where we will go. We will become aware of tiny, automatic movements as well as large, purposeful ones. We will see movement as metabolism, as action toward a goal, as communication, as remembering, and as creative expression. All of these conscious movement moments can be bodyful. Awareness will not be categorized as a function of mind but as a function of sensory and motoric processing, so that sensory awareness becomes one of our greatest allies in the work of moving toward bodyful states.

When we centralize movement in this way, the concept of body oscillations emerges. Used frequently in physics, music, engineering, chemistry, and biology, *oscillation* describes anything that moves back and forth in a regular manner, like vibrations or pulsations. The assertion of this book is that oscillation, this ability to move adaptively along a continuum of action, protects against polarization (being stuck in an extreme) and that overcoming polarizations promotes not only organismic health but also bodyfulness.

I will take a stand for this word *bodyful* as a separate and important construct in our cultivation of a conscious, contemplative, creative, and contributive life. To say *bodyful* reclaims a word box we have gradually lost as we developed and evolved as human beings. Repurposing words can help reclaim status and empowerment for oppressed peoples (such as *queer* and *gay*) or dignify power differentials (saying *administrative assistant* instead of *secretary*). Similarly, using the word *bodyful* may be as much a political act as a literary or poetic device.

This issue is about coming home. The body isn't a thing we have but an experience we are. Bodyfulness is about working toward our potential as a whole human animal that breathes as well as thinks, moves as well as sits still, takes action as well as considers, and exists not just because it thinks but because it dances, stretches, bounces, gazes, focuses, and attunes to others.

A Lived Context

I came to this word *bodyfulness* slowly and experientially. It began in my living room when I was about six years old, as I danced for my parents and their friends one evening. The look of tension and disapproval on their faces as they silently watched me jump and wiggle was so shaming that I stopped dancing entirely until I was a cultural anthropology student at the University of California, Los Angeles (UCLA), when out of a desperate need for a required arts elective that had to be on Tuesday and Thursday mornings, I took a modern dance class. Within weeks my world was upended. As I stretched and gestured and moved across the hardwood floors, it was as if I *re-membered* (re-embodied) myself. I certainly recognized myself for the first time in a long time. I "came out," not so much as a dancer but as a purposeful, conscious mover.

From that time forward I danced as well as academically studied the healing powers of movement, becoming a licensed professional counselor with board certifications as both a dance therapist and a body psychotherapist. I have clinically practiced body- and movement-based psychotherapy for over thirty-five years, privately and in hospital settings, as well as written two books, *Getting Our Bodies Back* and *Getting in Touch*.

In 1980 I moved to Boulder, Colorado, and got a full-time teaching job at Naropa University, founded by the Tibetan monk Chögyam Trungpa Rinpoche, where the faculty, students, and staff apply nonsectarian contemplative principles and practices to higher education. I found myself in an academic and scholarly setting that also valued wakefulness, contemplation, and compassionate action. Over time something ineffable in this environment seeped into me, and that something was mindfulness. Slowly this time, my world turned and again oriented in a right direction. Contemplative practice and being a teacher and researcher in higher education were the last missing elements, the pieces of the puzzle that brought everything into a coherent and refined clarity. Both mindfulness and bodyfulness were and continue to be essential to my sense of being a "full" self.

Life at the Margins

My six-year-old dancing disaster was neither unique nor particularly remarkable, but it was pivotal. It vividly marked the moment when I joined the ranks of the majority of people who feel shame when they view or directly experience their body. Body shame is so rampant in the United States, for instance, that nine out of ten people, when shown a silhouette of their body, will have a negative emotional response. Interestingly, this negative feeling occurs independently of what the person weighs. Research shows that in most developed countries we tend to internalize a shame-based image of our bodies fairly early and fairly enduringly.[4] Part of what I will propose in this book is that this internalized "somatophobia" results from most of us growing up in cultures or subcultures that reinforce *bodylessness*.

From the time that we humans began to sharpen our wits we began to dull our senses. The marginalization of the body has such a long and cross-cultural history that we barely notice or care that the oppression of our bodily selves is constant, insidious, and potentially devastating. We can see this in two ways: (1) in the historical use of physical difference as a weapon in the oppression and persecution of individuals and whole populations; and (2) in the devaluing of the body itself as a source of identity and authoritative knowledge about our direct, lived experience of ourselves and the world. In this context, both embodiment and bodyfulness are not something we can afford to marginalize any longer.

As technology becomes increasingly complex and crucial to modern living, the urge to keep overvaluing thoughts and ideas increases as the need for—and valuing of—physical labor decreases. Nielsen ratings note that in the United States both children and adults spend an average of over six hours a day sitting still in front of some kind of screen or monitor. Yearly, we are not only exercising less but also simply moving around less, and our remaining movements become more rote and routine. It seems timely that we attend to a body that increasingly gets neglected, devalued, and misused.

On top of the neglect of the body, modern society's new racism, classism, ableism, sexism, and ageism, may be increasingly enacted through the politics of the body. By indoctrinating us with narratives that valorize thin, light-skinned, young, fit, and able bodies, a second layer of disembodiment captures most of us sooner or later and wreaks havoc with our bodyfulness. In order to fully understand bodyfulness, this book will also examine the personal, social, and political issues around bodylessness.

How the Book Unfolds

This book begins, in part 1, by looking at the body itself—what it is, how it works, and what amazing stories the flesh can tell. The way the body works parallels the way the world works: via layers of networked systems that work best when they coregulate each other. The first part creates a context for bodyfulness in daily life as well as contemplative life by diving into the structural, functional, and symbolic nature of being a living organism. So many scientific, philosophical, and spiritual writings tell us about the nature of the mind—how it works and how it goes wrong—often equating it with our essential self. The body, however, tends to be described mechanistically in anatomy books or as an abstract concept in philosophical texts. When we are disembodied in this way, we live at a distance from the power and intelligence inherent in physical form, instead opting for the supremacy of an immaterial self, one we can never quite literally grasp.

The first two chapters of this book will take a different approach, seeing our physical structures—from cells to the whole body—as the essential self. We will look at the form and function of the body, both as a way to appreciate its intricacies as well as a means of reclaiming a sense of identity as an organism. This will involve, in chapter 1, working with eight principles of bodyfulness:

1. oscillation
2. balance
3. feedback loops
4. energy conservation
5. discipline
6. change and challenge
7. contrast through novelty
8. associations and emotions

Then, in chapter 2, we will look in a fresh way at the actual structures and functions of the body, from its cells to its tissues, organs, and systems, to understand them not just as names and locations but as living enactments of bodyfulness themes.

Part 2 develops the practice of bodyfulness by exploring four central themes:

1. breathing
2. sensing
3. moving
4. relating

These four body processes form the infrastructure of bodyfulness practices, and we will take time to explore each one as a means of constructing practices that develop and refine bodyfulness. They provide the means through which we can increase our wakefulness and make our actions more conscious and contributive.

Part 3 looks at how engagement with sensation, breath, movement, and relationship form an alchemical blend that can be understood as activism, not just in personal and political terms but also in contemplative ones. This part stresses the inherent practicality and playfulness in bodyfulness and asks us to make use of these elements in both simple and sophisticated ways. This involves understanding how the body changes itself, as well as how negative body experiences can interfere with bodyfulness. In this part I put the body into a more social context to show how disembodiment and bodylessness form so much of our inherited legacy. Activism, like oppression and marginalization, is enacted through and within our body; this part of the book invites us all to work with this practice more deeply, potentially restructuring and refining our definition of activism as well as nourishing our own sense of bodyful activism. In this way we can more confidently initiate and bring forward the changes we want for ourselves and our communities.

All chapters have experiential reflection exercises embedded throughout and many conclude with chapter practices. These exercises—drawn from existing traditions as well as developed by me, others, or you—are all designed to help you reclaim a bodyful life. Therapists, teachers, and counselors may also want to use these practices with clients and students, at their discretion. The exercises alternate between freestanding or embedded, structured and unstructured. In other words, some exercises are meant to be done on their own, as a dedicated time of practice. Other exercises coach you in the art of embedding a practice such as conscious breathing into daily living—while in a stressful meeting, during a tender exchange with a friend, or at a bus stop. Both embodiment and bodyfulness, in this sense, take place as stand-alone activities and as ones that weave themselves into each moment. They can also be cultivated by trusted practices that have been handed down over time by various traditions, and by spontaneous actions that just feel right in the moment and draw from the authority and activism of your living body. Please alter them to suit yourself, trusting that you know best what your limits and interests are. Stop any exercise that becomes unmanageable. Having a strong reaction to an exercise, whether physical, emotional, or cognitive, is a sign that you might best find a professional with whom to further explore them. They are suggestions and guidances, and only you know the delicate and changing balance between what may be too challenging and not challenging enough.

At the end of the book you will find an "Additional Notes and References" section. This section includes publishing information for sources mentioned throughout the book, cites sources, and briefly explains more technical details of concepts you might be curious about. It also includes further resources and references concerning the topics, people, and practices cited in the chapters.

Because I'm an academic as well as a therapist and value critical thinking as well as conscious moving, I have written this book so that you can relate to the material on multiple levels. The philosophy, psychology, and social theory connected with bodyfulness weave their way throughout the chapters, while at the same time inviting you to pause and reflect on or experience directly your body and its movements, sensations, breathing, and relationships to other bodies. The book is designed to be read from start to finish, in order, but trust your judgment about how you use it. For instance, you could read it through in order, or you could read each chapter's discussions first, then go through the book again and just work with the exercises. The discussions and exercises are each designed to build cumulatively, so it might be best to start with them at the beginning and work through to the end. Bodyfulness involves discipline, as any contemplative practice does, and this discipline expresses itself via thinking, feeling, and moving with what you are doing, including reading this book. Let yourself explore how you want to read this book in a bodyful way!

I hope that this book is a resource for you and that by practicing bodyfulness you in turn can be a resource for your loved ones, your community, and your society. May we all live consciously, joyfully, and intentionally, our bodily selves waking, moving, and working together.

Chapter Practices

- Most of us have a favorite stretch, a simple yoga pose, or a specific way that we take a few breaths as a means to take care of ourselves, reduce stress, and promote our health. We repeat these practices we have formally or informally learned because they feel right and do the trick. Go ahead and do one of them now, just for a minute. As you do, focus your attention on the act itself. Practice locating your attention where the action is—in what you are doing physically. Bodyfulness begins to develop when you pay attention to what your physical form is experiencing and doing, even in familiar activities. Practice shining a beam of attention toward the surface and interior of your body and letting it land on strong sensory signals as well as subtler ones and areas where there doesn't seem to be any sensory signal at all. Work at simply observing your body in the activity, pushing back against the urge to explain or judge what you are doing, or think about something else. Just stay present with the action for a minute or two.

- Find a comfortable position—it could be standing, sitting, or lying down. Close your eyes and simply pay attention to sensations within your body for a few minutes. It could be sensations of pressure, temperature, tension, hunger, fullness, tingling—anything. Begin to notice what comes up as you attend to your body. Does your attention get pulled to certain types of sensations, such as pleasurable or painful ones? Does it get pulled to certain areas of your body? No problem, just note that. When you feel ready, work at putting your attention on a part of your body that you weren't tracking before, an area such as your elbow or chin, where you might not have been getting any signals. Just rest your attention there for a few moments, even if you don't seem to be getting any sensory reading from it. Often parts of the body go to sleep a bit when they don't get much attention, so sensations may or may not show up as you attend to these areas. If you are interested, you might want to repeat the exercise in a different position. The difference between standing, sitting, and lying down, for instance, can generate different bodily experiences.

• As you read this book, take a few small moments here and there to turn your attention from the page and notice your body. Notice your position. Are you still comfortable? Notice your energy level. Is it time for a break, where you might eat or drink something, or move around a bit? Notice your breathing. Is it easy and flowing? Make any adjustments that your body signals you to make, and then go back to reading—or not!

PART ONE

The Body of Bodyfulness

1

The Eight Core Principles of Bodyfulness

W HEN WE REFLECT on the nature of the body, two basic themes arise: what bodies actually are and who we are as bodies. The dictionary lists a number of definitions of *body*, but one that may be useful here is the notion that the body is the main or central part of anything, like the body of a play or a book. Our body can be defined as the center of who we are as well as how others perceive us and interact with us. From the perspective of being a *body*, we are a process, a moving symphony of breathing, digesting, respirating, thinking, feeling. Our body is also tangible. We have weight, solidity, shape, and size, and because of this we can look to the physical sciences for guidance. Physics, for instance, might say that our body is both matter and energy. We have mass, and this mass produces and consumes energy as a function of being alive; that is, we move around under our own power. (Inanimate objects can only move when something else moves them.) Self-initiated movement defines the difference between being animate and inanimate, and between life and death—in death our heart stops moving, our lungs stop moving, our brain cells stop generating electrical waves. So, once again, to speak about our body is to speak about movement. Let's familiarize ourselves with eight principles of movement that create the scaffolding for bodyfulness.

Principle 1: Oscillation

As we noted before, one of the most elemental movements that occurs in nature is oscillation. Everything that has mass oscillates, from subatomic particles to whole organisms. Oscillation involves going back and forth between two positions or states, back and forth across some point of equilibrium. Think waves on the shore or a pendulum swinging. Oscillation is a complete movement, whether it's up and down, side to side, or forward and back. The body oscillates constantly: our heart expands and contracts (heartbeats) and generates oscillatory waves of electromagnetic pulses, our breath goes in and out (breathing), our brain cells generate their own electromagnetic pulses (brain waves), our muscles tense and relax (tonus) and generate electromagnetic waves, our digestive tract contracts and then releases (peristalsis). These oscillations repeat on the cellular level as well, an example being ion gates opening and closing to let chemicals in and out of cells.

Our body oscillates, all the way from our cells to our whole body moving forward and back, left to right, up and down. In the next chapters we will look at how these oscillations contribute to health or illness on physical, emotional, cognitive, and contemplative levels. For now, we can assume that they figure into bodyfulness in literal and symbolic ways. Cooperating with our natural oscillations may be one of our best means of developing a bodyful self.

For example, as any back-and-forth movement occurs, the arc of this movement creates a continuum, let's say from left to right. Moving back and forth along a continuum may have important symbolic value, calling to mind the idea that at the limits of a continuum we experience extremes and that the middle is often a place where we feel more grounded and tend to find equanimity. Buddhism calls this the Middle Path. For our health's sake, we are enjoined to eat and drink in moderation, for instance. In psychotherapy and counseling we talk about clients consistently experiencing extreme states and how damaging this can be to their ongoing well-being. We can define mental and emotional illness as an inability to let go of extreme states or an overuse or inappropriate use of them. If we can't stop being angry, for instance, we tend to experience everyday events as defensive emergencies.

This metaphor of continuums applies to social systems as well. We often call people on the extreme political left or right as the "lunatic fringe." Being stuck in extremes, we often demonize the other extreme on the continuum and then become polarized. When polarization happens, paralysis and aggression ensue. When we move within and along continuums, physics dictates that we spend the bulk of our time moving within the middle zone of that range.

From the principle of oscillation, we can see bodyfulness as involving an ability to consciously move along many different arcs, oscillating widely along a continuum of actions and states, such as from hard work to deep rest, from solitude to sociality, from self-care to the care of others, or from rare extremes to common conditions. Oscillatory movement, rather than fixed positions, can be what facilitates a sense of balance and equanimity. Bodyfulness involves the ability to navigate adaptively through the changing circumstances of life as consciously and gracefully as possible.

Practice for Oscillation

Take a moment now to check in with your breathing, just noticing its back-and-forth, back-and-forth. See if you can track your heart beating (you can put a finger on your wrist or the side of your neck to help you listen). Notice what images, memories, feelings, words come up as you simply attend to these organismic oscillations in your body.

Principle 2: Balance

Bodyfulness also involves balancing, the ability to poise oneself within certain states, much like the ability to stand for a bit on one leg, a literal skill that is critical for the development of core body tone, which in turn protects us against falls and accidents. Literally, our body also needs to hover around certain metabolic set points, such as 98.6 degrees Fahrenheit for internal body temperature. We also have fairly narrow set points for such things as blood sugar, blood pressure, cholesterol, and acidity/alkalinity. Deviating from these set points can be dangerous to our health, and this is why modern medicine monitors them, medicates them, and enjoins us to live our lives close to them.

In many meditation traditions, we learn the skill of evenly hovering attention or concentration on one thing. We balance our mental focus at one point and work toward increasing our ability to stay there, standing on one mental leg, so to speak, until it increases our core contemplative fitness. This skill of concentration, done with minimal effort and without judgment, can have many beneficial effects. These same meditation traditions examine at length the concept of stillness, which occurs when we can easily hold our attention for sustained periods of time, much like standing on one leg quietly, without having to wave our arms around. It's this athleticism of the act of attending, more than the content of what we do or don't pay attention to, that matters. In stillness we quiet the discursive mind, we listen to a kind of inner silence that can be powerfully transformative. Yet the body teaches us that relative stillness and balance occur as a result of ongoing, tiny movement oscillations. We will talk about this more deeply in subsequent chapters, but for now we can bookmark the concept of balance as being a component of bodyfulness, whether that balancing involves hopping on one leg or finding an overall sense of balance in one's life.

Oscillating between balancing in one place and traveling through space, between being and doing, may be the ultimate key. We work, we rest. We inhale, we exhale. We go it alone, we seek out company. As the Bible states in Ecclesiastes 3:4, "For everything there is a season, a time for every matter under the heavens . . . a time to mourn and a time to dance." Oscillating and balancing literally keeps us alive and well. Oscillating consciously in our relationships also promotes the conditions for bodyfulness.

Practice for Balance

If you can, take a few minutes to play with standing on one leg, then the other. One leg might be easier than the other. Notice what sensations you feel, what images or memories come up, what thoughts arise. For now, just notice.

Principle 3: Feedback Loops

Another extension of the principles of oscillation and balance has to do with the body's penchant for feedback loops. Every part of us sends and receives information to every other part of us, constantly, as a means of coordinating actions for the good of the whole. Some neuroscientists, such as Candace Pert, think of the mind as the circulating flow of information throughout the body and our nerves and blood vessels as major highways conducting that flow. Chapter 2 will explore some of our most cherished physical highways, also called feedback loops. One way to understand the relationship between the thinking part of the brain and the rest of the body, however, is to imagine a feedback loop that runs bottom up and top down. Top-down processing implies using one's verbal and cognitive reflections to promote behavioral change—our head talking to our body. We can, at times, talk ourselves out of a bad idea, for instance, or feel freed by a thoughtful realization about an issue. This is the basis of the psychoanalyst Sigmund Freud's "talking cure," the idea that cognitive insight can trickle down to a change in behavior. It also forms the basis of many sitting meditation practices, for instance, in which we work to create gaps between thoughts.

At other times we can use bottom-up processing by working with our behavior directly, invoking the "just do it" (or don't do it) strategy; our bodily behavior then changes how and what we think. This is the basis for getting your butt to the gym, since reflecting on your physical fitness won't change it. It also demonstrates why body-centered contemplative practices, such as yoga or tai chi, can bring about improvements in thought and mood. This bottom-up process also involves the direct emotional and relational body-to-body exchanges that occur between people, such as a therapist's compassionate gaze, a parent's ability to distinguish between their baby's different cries, or a friend putting their hand on their heart in response to you saying something emotionally potent. These oscillatory, wordless body exchanges have been shown to be extremely effective in repairing old relational wounds because they give people a direct experience of feeling emotionally connected and understood. We will look at this a bit more in chapter 9.

Ideally this bottom-up/top-down feedback loop works as a single unit, producing regulated states within us as well as good connections in relationships. Errors in one mode can be checked by the other. For instance, we can think from the top down that we are not frightened, but our sweaty palms and dilated pupils belie that. Or we can bottom-up reach for a piece of cake, and our thoughts can remind us that the last time we did this we got a stomachache.

Top-down and bottom-up processing modes are implicated in many major life issues, such as addiction, mental illness, emotional regulation, relational bonding, and others. This is because sensory nerves always, sooner or later, hook up to motor nerves, which is to say that sensations always ask for a response, an action, a movement. If symptoms are honored and dealt with, they tend to subside. If they are ignored or suppressed, they tend to scream louder or stop sending the signal (even though the cause of the symptom persists). In either case, the movement response fails to coordinate and cooperate with the sensation and an important feedback loop breaks, setting us up for illnesses at multiple levels. Contemplative practices help us break this cycle of suffering. In bodyfully oriented contemplative moments, we are reminded that practice becomes whole-bodied when it includes and connects our physical, emotional, and mental states. In this book we will keep looking into this important feedback loop.

Practice for Feedback Loops

- *Starting from the top down.* Pick a part of your body that currently exhibits some small symptom, such as tension or achiness. Take a few minutes to put your attention there without trying to change it. Just notice; resist judging or explaining it. Then think about this symptom for a few minutes from a top-down perspective, not feeling that you have to come to a specific conclusion but just putting your mind to it in an open and curious way. Notice what ideas come up, whether they be problem focused or solution focused. Take the ideas under advisement, treating them like hypotheses that you might want to test either by devising an experiment or by consulting others who may have some knowledge about this.

- *Starting from the bottom up.* Now pay attention to the sensations of the symptom itself, the physical details of it. Sensations are signals, and from a bottom-up perspective we can work with them directly. This time, play with the hypothesis that this sensation might be a movement that is being held in, held back, or held down. Take a few minutes to check back in with the details of the symptom. Instead of imposing a mental solution, work to allow that part of your body to make small movements that are not about relieving the symptom but rather telling its story through moving it. For instance, if the symptom is tightness, let it tighten more because that is what it's already doing or saying. If it aches, how would you let your body express the ache directly? Nothing fancy, just let that part of your body move a bit, without explanation but with lots of caring attention.

Principle 4: Energy Conservation

The body, like all physical systems, operates with limited resources. We only have so much energy, and if demand for it in the short run is high, the body will turn off certain metabolic processes and give that energy savings to whatever activity is deemed more important. For example, if we are in danger, our body turns off digestion, immune system activities, and reproductive metabolism in order to give more energy to fight or flight. This rerouting of energy resources is critical for our short-term survival, yet if we feel stressed or threatened frequently, the chronic activation of this same mechanism can damage our ability to digest properly, to ward off illness, or to make babies.

Another way the body conserves energy on an ongoing basis is to form habits. Habits start out as conscious actions that are practiced enough times that they become automatic and habitual, and automatic actions are *a lot* less consumptive of energy. Consciousness is *very* metabolically expensive, and we try to reserve it for what we have learned to deem as important to pay attention to right now. Take a minute to remember the act of learning something, such as riding a bike. In the beginning you were very vigilant, monitoring all the variables involved—balancing, braking, steering, pedaling, navigating—all at once. Initially this was likely overwhelming and tiring. It takes time and conscious practice before biking becomes routine and "easy." Habits are a blessing and a curse because of this. It's a real blessing that, after spending some expensive, conscious time learning how to steer, lean, brake, and pedal, we can get on a bike and ride across town without much attention to the process at all. We can even turn our consciousness to talking, looking at the view, or figuring out traffic, while our body practices the automatic habit in the background. This physical capacity for multitasking occurs constantly. We are always engaging in many physical things at once, only a few of which we are actively monitoring.

The curse part of habits comes into play when we practice things that are no longer good for us or are inherently bad for us. Contemplative traditions often speak of their practices as confronting and dissolving habits of mind, such as the tendency to ruminate, judge, or compartmentalize. Another way of making new habits is psychotherapy, which sees itself as surfacing stored, automatic schemas, emotions, and tendencies that no longer serve us and using the hard, conscious work of reflection and insight to leverage therapeutic change. Imagine a child growing up in a family experiencing domestic violence, where yelling was usually followed by hitting. This child likely learned to cower and freeze whenever voices got loud. As an adult, this body habit repeats with any loud voice, even joyful shouts at a baseball game. Our body habits are like movement memories; they represent predispositions to move and react in certain ways, a kind of *body box* that can confine and confuse us. We often lament that we don't have enough "willpower" to get out of these body boxes. Yet the principle of energy conservation shows us that using our will to overcome an ingrained habit can be more complex than we thought.

From a bodyfulness perspective, practice involves surfacing our body's habits—woven in with thought and emotional habits—and generating new options via conscious breathing, moving, sensing, and relating to others. Just willfully telling ourselves to change won't be enough. Change tends to be expensive because it requires both consciousness and behavioral effort to overcome the habit. Some people are dubbed "change resistant." However, we can appreciate that change can simply be too expensive for them, given how much energy they are expending elsewhere for other purposes, such as self-defense or just trying to make the rent. It takes relative safety, courage, and energy to change, yet the results are worth it once these conditions are present. Hopefully we will all work for the social good, so that the conditions for change are accessible to all. In this way good mental, emotional, and physical habits can be a conservation blessing, freeing us up for a more creative and contributive life.

Practice for Energy Conservation

Next time you brush your teeth, change it up a bit, perhaps brushing with your nondominant hand. This is *not* about training yourself to brush your teeth differently but rather an exercise in noticing how wonderful automatic body habits can be. You experience how discombobulating it can be to flummox your habits and how much attention and energy you need to use in order to flummox them and still get your teeth brushed. The advanced practice here is to notice patterns of any daily activity, such as walking or eating. In certain cases, such as chronic injury, you may need to deconstruct some of these body habits—the body has learned to be injured—and lay down different ones. It can be a lot of work, which is why we sometimes feel reluctant to make the change. Self-compassion, based in conscious breathing, moving, sensing, and relating to self, other, and the world, can give much of the energy for the task.

Principle 5: Discipline

In order to create and maintain physical habits that support physical, emotional, and cognitive well-being, we need to practice, and to practice we require discipline. *Discipline* is a word that can occupy some varied and dramatic word boxes. It can be associated with mastery, punishment, concentration, deprivation, devotion, and inquiry. What does a disciplined body mean to you? From a bodyfulness perspective, we want to play with and reflect on this question. From an anatomical perspective, discipline is about maximizing operational efficiency, which is related to energy conservation. Athletes Serena Williams and Michael Jordan make it look easy because it *is* easier for them after years of disciplined practice.

Another expression of the body's need to conserve energy is that it tends to lose capacity with things it hasn't been doing for a while. A muscle that isn't exercised will lose strength and therefore its ability to move efficiently. A cognitive capacity that isn't refreshed will erode over time. The body truly operates on a "use it or lose it" principle. This may be why all spiritual traditions as well as physical disciplines stress the importance of practice, practice, practice. They urge us to do things consciously so as to lay down new, automatic, healthy habits, and as a way to conserve energy with enough left over for the important things. And repeat and repeat. Make a new habit out of it. That habit will create bodily efficiencies that create a disciplined body, one that finds things easier to do.

Discipline likely underlies grace. When we first learn a new physical activity, whether it be hammering a nail or learning to swim, we at first feel clumsy and awkward. Our movements tend to be inefficient, and we often feel tired afterward. With practice, the movements become more graceful and more aesthetically satisfying. It's no wonder that the word *grace* describes both movement aesthetics and spiritual attainment.

Practice for Discipline

This is a thought reflection. You may want to jot down a few notes in the midst. On a day-to-day basis, what do you habitually practice? First think about the daily physical things that can be more obvious, such oral hygiene. (Yay for flossing!) Then move to the less obvious things, such as how you tend to look someone in the eye as you speak to them. Range widely in your daily life, recalling your automatic ways of being in the world in both bodyful and bodyless ways. We practice both good and bad habits throughout the day. Perhaps you "practice" a lot of TV watching or you are great at your yoga practice while you have a hard time with your money-spending practices. Take some time to assess what you tend to do repeatedly and automatically. Try not to judge yourself, just notice. Throughout this exercise, pay attention to what happens in your body when you contemplate making a particular habit more conscious, or more or less frequently practiced. Just notice, and work with what comes up in your awareness by holding it and caring for it.

Principle 6: Change and Challenge

A few decades ago, scientists began rethinking the idea that when we are little we develop by producing tons of new cells (called growing) that work hard and eventually create a mature organism, followed by at first a slow decline involving cell death slightly outpacing cellular regeneration. Eventually cell death accelerates and results in our death. For example, until recently neuroscientists believed that after about age twenty-five we didn't grow any new brain cells. The original thought was that adulthood was when all our capacities were fairly fixed, and we could just look forward to a slow but increasingly rapid decline. Then scientists discovered *neuroplasticity*. While it's still true that our somatic cells eventually wear out in ways that outstrip cellular repair and regeneration, we have found ample evidence that over our entire lifetime we can fundamentally change at the cellular level as a result of neuroplasticity. While the definition of this term restricts itself to nerve cells (neurons), the principle of plastic change likely occurs throughout the body as well. Change and even growth occur constantly and normally throughout our lives.

While the principle of discipline highlights the fact that we need to use it or will most likely lose it, it's also true that how we use it can change how it's structured and how it functions. Our direct experiences generate constant input to our brain and the rest of our body, and these inputs change how cells organize themselves inside us as well as how many of them there are to do their work. These inputs even turn on and off certain genes. The term *genetically determined* is being altered by research that shows that our lived experiences actually influence, on an ongoing basis, which genes turn on and express themselves and which ones don't. (The field of study concerned with this is called *epigenesis*.)

During different phases of development, another type of input involves "overproduction and pruning." Huge numbers of new neurons—way too many, actually—are produced in the brains of children as well as of adolescents. What happens is that our direct experiences—our behavior and actions—stimulate some of these new neurons to fire and connect with each other, while not stimulating others. The ones that are not used die off in order to conserve energy. This is how practice lays down new skills on a cellular level, via making some nerves and their connections to each other strengthen while others wither from lack of use. Aging likely involves a slowing down of the overproduction of new cells so that we have fewer and fewer new cells to work with in terms of changing our patterns of use. However, we are always producing new somatic cells.

As we get more familiar with bottom-up processing, we can see that change is quite literally a somatic experience. While we operate within genetic limitations, we are less limited than we previously thought. To a certain extent we can directly influence how many new cells we produce. We now know that we can learn new things during our entire life span and retain capacities longer, even into our advanced years. Our daily experiences determine how fully we can operate within these expanded genetic limits. How can we influence our capacity to continue to change and grow? The key word here is *challenge.* In order to change something, we must challenge the status quo. Bodyfulness involves artfully challenging our status quo.

The exercise at the end of this next section will cover principles 6 and 7.

Principle 7: Contrast Through Novelty

On a cellular level, learning something new entails growing new nerve cells as well as growing the connectivity between them, as we noted above. On a whole-body level, learning something new involves having experiences that challenge our programming.

Researchers have found that the learning process begins when the nervous system, which monitors our inner and outer environment largely below our awareness, senses a contrast. Something we are experiencing has changed, or something is new and unknown. This novelty wakes up certain parts of the brain, which then focus attention on the new stimuli and gather sensory data about that new thing. Is it safe? Incoming data, before we are ever aware of it, is first vetted to assess whether it's dangerous. It's next compared to our historical memory banks. Have we experienced this before? Is it familiar? If it's familiar, our nervous system tends to go down a "been there, done that" road, and we stop paying much attention to it (the neural basis for how familiar things can be taken for granted). But if it's unfamiliar, if it creates a contrast with what we are used to, then our conscious brain lights up and we start focusing our senses toward that new experience. We consciously take in the new experiential data, and if we feel sufficiently drawn to it or emotionally invested in it, we will commit this new experience to memory, which is another way of saying that we have just learned something. This also explains why we have difficulty learning things that we don't care about.

These understandings about learning by contrast formed the basis for Edmund Jacobson, a physician, to develop a practice called *progressive relaxation*. He noted that a person can relax a tense muscle much more deeply when they first tense it up more, creating sensory contrast, which wakes up and mobilizes the body to learn to let go.

A second theory concerning how we change emerges from this first understanding about learning. Simply put, if we keep operating the same way, we don't learn anything new. Learning occurs in atmospheres of mild to moderate challenge to the status quo. The developmental psychologist Lev Vygotsky called this the *zone of proximal development*, the zone we learn in because we are not resting in our comfort zone, but we are also not distressingly overwhelmed or too far outside our comfort zone. New experiences in the zone of proximal development are energy consuming, challenging as well as manageable, and are learned from. They can even be fun. This learning can stimulate new growth, structural and functional change in the body, and increased well-being. Increasingly, expending energy to challenge oneself to learn new things is seen as the key to healthy aging as well as the basis for therapeutic change. To overcome our strong and sensible interest in conserving energy, we also need to challenge ourselves. As the book progresses, we will return frequently to the twin concepts of contrast and challenge as essential components in bodyfulness.

Practice for Change, Challenge, Contrast, and Novelty

- Open up a dictionary and find a word you don't know the meaning of. Read the definition and practice the word in a sentence so you learn it. Notice at the same time how your body is handling this activity. Is it alert, calm, hypervigilant? Notice what associations arise as you learn the first word. Now put your body in a kind of goofy position that you don't usually put yourself in, while you find and learn a second word. Have fun putting your new word into a sentence while in your goofy position. In a few weeks check back in to see how you have remembered (or not) the new words. What was the relationship between the goofy position and the ability to remember each of the words? Hint: goofy can equate with novelty and with being more alert and involved in the learning.

- Take a minute to see if you can recall a time when you felt stuck or frustrated when trying to learn something or an old dream where you were trying to do something but you just couldn't, such as trying to talk but no sound came out, trying to run away but your feet wouldn't cooperate, or taking a calculus test having never taken the class. Notice how your body feels as you remember the attempt at learning or the dream. These remembrances may be a kind of facing into what it's like to be overwhelmed by something you can't do or don't know how to do. Notice how your present, awake body processes this recollection. Work to just hold this response with your caring and noninterpretive attention.

Principle 8: Associations and Emotions

We noted that when the nervous system receives incoming sensory data, it associates or compares these sensations to our memory stores and then determines if we care about it, all before and below our conscious awareness of the experience. *Caring*, another word for our emotional experiencing of something, is so foundational to our well-being that the body begins to emotionally process incoming events automatically, outside our control and below our consciousness. By the time we are old enough to remember specific events, we have already stored myriad emotional memories about whether or not the world is basically safe, whether or not people can be trusted, or whether or not experimentation and play are worth it. And our body moves in the world accordingly.

The brain constantly forms associations so that memories—emotional, physical, and cognitive—can guide our future actions. We can directly experience this associative infrastructure when we daydream. We might start out with a visual memory of our grandma's front porch, then shift to an olfactory memory of the smell of her cooking collard greens coming through the window screen. Yum! Then we remember that we forgot to buy spinach for dinner, and then it goes to last night's dinner table where we had a fight with our sister. Yuck! At any one transition the reverie could go in a different direction—the smell coming through the screen could bring up a memory of a broken window screen at home you keep forgetting to fix. The associations tend to ride on waves of feeling. Associations are another type of body signal, this time from the emotional unconscious. Listening to these wordless signals can in some cases give you higher-quality information about a problem than trying to think it through.

Sigmund Freud was the first clinician to understand this process in a way that could be leveraged for therapeutic change. He called it *free association*, where he would ask clients to start talking and keep talking to see what came up. What often comes up are buried associations (emotional memories) that can be worked with to bring about psychological change. In practicing bodyfulness we will take advantage of this natural process of forming associations on waves of feeling. We will learn to practice *physical free association* as a way to access emotional connections that drive our behavior.

The word *emotion* literally means "to move out"—e-motion. First, before we are conscious of a stimulus, we associate the stimulus to stored emotional memories. Then, still before we are aware of it, we set up a response. Emotions organize, shape, and enable our actions in response to a stimulus; this is called emotional processing. We only become aware of an emotion *as* we are about to act on it. If we have what is called *executive control*, we can consciously decide whether to move according to the emotion or inhibit the movement. Two-year-olds are famous for tantrums because their brains are not mature enough to exert executive control over their emotions. Caregivers function as external executive controls—"No, you may not bite your brother"—while the child internalizes enough disciplined experiences to organize their own executive control over the urge to bite.

Emotions move us from the bottom up. Our top-down processes help to shape, allow, inhibit, and enable our emotions to either become enemies or friends in our daily lives. Bodyfulness practices will take advantage of this movement principle as a means of helping our emotions be our friends.

Practice for Associations and Emotions

We have actually been working with this principle already, so let's see how we can expand on it. The trick is to find associations to things rather than explanations for them. Start with a mildly distressing memory. Take some time to remember the incident in descriptive detail. As you do so, notice what comes up in your direct experience. Do you get an image of your brother when you remember that trip to a farm when you were five? Do you get a queasy feeling in your stomach when you recall almost getting hit by a car when crossing the street a few weeks ago? Associations are often related to sensations, so they arise as sounds, images, smells, tensions, related memories, or emotions. They don't necessarily seem related to what you are remembering. Just let the associations come without trying to categorize them or take meaning from them. Make sure to pay close attention to associations that come up in the body, such as sensations, changes of arousal, or small movements. Welcome them.

Now switch to a mildly pleasurable memory and practice the same exercise. This exercise can be just as important as working with distress, as many of us have learned to limit or be fearful of our positive experiences.

Putting the Principles Together

Together these eight elements can be regarded as the precepts that govern bodyfulness. They arise from our contemplations of how the literal body structures itself and functions in the world. Our body, with its freedom to change as well as its mortal limitations, teaches us how we can occupy bodyful states. By engaging with oscillations, balances, feedback loops, energy conservation, discipline, change and challenge, contrast and novelty, and associations and emotions, we build a foundation for bodyfulness practices.

All eight principles share movement as their common and unifying theme. Oscillation reminds us that finding our home base involves moving along continuums and that our home base can change. Balance illustrates that stillness requires poised efforts on micro levels. Feedback loops keep us balanced by integrating the movement of thoughts and sensations with the movements of the body in action. Energy conservation provides us with perspective on our limited energy resources and orients us to consider how we can use our resources in the service of grace and efficiency. We can achieve that grace and efficiency through understanding and practicing disciplined movement—a gentle stretch, a timely nap, or a brisk walk. When we want or need to change, we can appreciate that this means we will move outside our comfort zone, where we can harness novelty to help ourselves wake up and guide our new efforts. Lastly, we can make use of the natural movements of emotions and the associations that arise with them as a way to access the energy and the motivation we need to move in and navigate a complex world.

Subsequent chapters continue this oscillation between the literal nature of the body and the useful metaphors that literalness can suggest. In this way, the body shows itself to be the main or central part of who we are, individually and collectively, in ways that can reduce our fears, promote our well-being, and help us lead a bodyful life.

Chapter Practices

- At points in the day when you are about to make a decision, especially a small one, take a moment to check in with your body sensations before making your choice. For instance, if you are choosing between staying a bit longer at a friend's house or leaving for home, take a moment to just listen to the small goings-on inside. The sensations you notice—such as a clenching in the gut when you imagine leaving for home now—may feel like a strong signal that will help you make the decision, or they may just feel like random inner experiences. Don't try to be psychic and interpret an itchy arm as one thing or another. Just get used to listening to your body before and during the decision-making process. The more you listen, the more you will learn about how your body might be "moving with" your choices. This will grow your authoritative knowledge of your body and your emotional intelligence.

- *A five- to ten-minute practice.* Sit comfortably. Take a few minutes to purposefully oscillate your attention from inside to outside your body. When your attention goes in, just notice different sensations, no matter whether they are pleasurable, neutral, or painful, loud, or quiet. When you feel ready, oscillate your attention out and visually notice your surroundings. In a relaxed manner, land your eyes on various objects in the room or outdoors. It doesn't matter what you pay attention to; the practice is about noticing this flow of attention in and out. You don't need to split the time fifty-fifty, just notice what it's like to oscillate your attention. Notice if any preferences or reactions come up. Do you prefer to be more in or more out? Does one condition feel a bit safer? More familiar? Just take note of these patterns of attention.

- Whenever it comes to your attention in the next few days, stop what you are doing for a few moments and pay attention to the inner goings-on of your body. As much as possible, feel the subtle signals it's constantly producing: pressure here, tingling there, small ache just there. Take a moment to notice these things, and work to refrain from thinking anything about them. Try not to interpret the sensations, just listen to them without preference, and notice any associations that occur as a result of listening to them. You may notice that some areas are sensory hot spots and others seem like deserts, where very little is going on. We have more sensory neurons in some areas of our body than others. We can train ourselves over time to ignore some areas and enrich others (neuroplasticity), likely as a result of being told to, from conscious practices such as those associated with learning to play musical instruments, or from efforts to enhance pleasure or avoid pain. That makes sense. But for now, just work at making every sensation equal in your attention, with no judgment or even explanation. This will help you dehabituate your body awareness, to confront old habits that cause you to ignore some parts of your body or get obsessed by others.

- This exercise pushes back against our tendency to create interpretations and judgments about our body, an action that obstructs bodyfulness. See if you can notice instances during the day when you criticize your body or the bodies of others (either out loud or in your head). When we become a critic, we make a thumbs-up or a thumbs-down toward ourselves or others. So critiquing bodies involves judging them to be either good or bad. What can be important here is learning to tell the difference between loving and caring for your body and evaluating it as a kind of object. The difference may sound like "I feel good today" or "I like the way I look today" versus "My hips are too big" or "My figure is better than hers." Just notice this critiquing—it's frequency, patterns, focus, associated feelings—but don't try to change it right now. Just observe the details of doing it. You might want to make the mental statement, "I notice I'm critiquing my body/others' bodies right now."

2

The Anatomy of Bodyfulness

KNOWLEDGE IS POWER. The aim of this chapter is to help us learn about our body in a meaningful way. More than just memorizing the words for body parts and their functions, we can re-member ourselves as a bodyfulness project, as a way to prepare ourselves for the wisdom and teachings of the body. This examination of our literal form can be like studying a template and can help us bring bodyfulness to life. This knowing begins when we look at the different levels of organization that compose our body, starting with the cell and working up to the entire organism. At each level, contemplative concepts such as interdependence, the middle path, oscillation, exchange, and permeability will be visible. Again, we will alternate between the literal and the metaphoric as a means of appreciating different ways of knowing the body. We will also oscillate between metaphors that are handed down to us by culture and family, as well as notice metaphoric associations that arise spontaneously as we work with our body in the present moment.

Cells

Our first bodyful contemplation is that of the cell, the smallest unit of life.

In the beginning there were stem cells, those wonderful I-could-be-anything-when-I-grow-up packets of possibility. We get the term *stem* from the fact that these basic, undifferentiated cells generate every specific cell in the body, eventually composing the whole organism. Another way to put it is that we begin as one—a unified, undifferentiated existence—holding the potential for human form but not yet expressing it. Biology calls these original cells *totipotent*, able to become anything in the body.

After just a few rounds of cell division postfertilization, these totipotent fetal stem cells start the process of creating the entire body, self-renewing indefinitely, replicating not only new second-generation stem cells but also cells that are specific types: muscle, bone, nerve, and so forth. The second-generation stem cells—called pluripotent, meaning able to be many things but not all things—huddle deep in the body, mostly in bone marrow and the intestines, and work to repair and regenerate the body at the cellular level. These second-generation stem cells are more specialized and therefore more limited. The stem cells in the gut can only generate more gut lining, for instance.

By far the greatest number of cells generated in later divisions—called somatic cells; *soma* in Greek means "body"—become specific things, committing at their outset to being one type of cell: blood, heart, fingernail. Because of their specific identity, somatic cells will wear out, get sick, and die, ultimately causing our death as an individual. Somatic cells, unlike stem cells, are programmed to die and are continuously replaced, some faster than others. For instance, our skin cells wear out quickly and are renewed about every thirty days, while some bone cells can take years to be replaced. On a cellular level, our death is often a process of somatic cell death outstripping cell birth (very common in the brain). Stem cells might be the metaphorical equivalent of living in the Garden of Eden, and somatic cells represent our exit from Eden into earthly life and death.

Contemplative metaphors abound in stem and somatic cells. What can we see about the nature of our identity when we learn that we start out undifferentiated and "totally potent," but with a promise to become many different but interdependent elements that are very specific? And when that promise is fulfilled and we become someone in particular, with very particular eyes, arms, and ears, we lock in both our sense of individual identity and our death. In the cell is where we can first understand the Buddhist notion that we are a self and a no-self. We are everything (or nothing) and something in particular. When we die, our somatic and stem cells die, yet some of our stem cells have generated gametes (sperm or ovum), and some of them might have "mated" with other stem cells from someone else, producing totipotent stem cells that created another body, itself containing and generating both stem and somatic cells. Our myriad, mortal somatic cells got many of us to the place where we could blend our stem cells with someone else's. They also interdependently tended and nurtured our totipotent and pluripotent cells/selves our whole lives. Life goes on. Cells go on. Deathless cells can only be so because of the support of cells that die, and vice versa.

Regardless of whether our stem cells and somatic cells cooperate to help generate children, our bodies *are* totipotent, pluripotent, and of limited potency. We may blame and fear the body because it so obviously sickens and dies, yet it can only do so. This specific somatic self is our only means of holding and caring for our totipotent cells/selves. Our mortal body in this sense is our means of cradling and expressing our less limited bodily self. How we live our life *now* in ways that embody and express all levels of our potency may be a physical template for how we understand enlightenment, or what some call self-realization or a state of grace.

Peering into the structure of any cell, whether stem or somatic, we find further bodyful metaphors. Every cell encircles itself with a cell wall, called a membrane, that encloses and protects the important stuff within. The cell wall ensures the cell's integrity by keeping its inner ingredients in close proximity so that they can easily influence each other and cause cellular metabolism to occur. The results of those metabolic processes that use enzymes, proteins, hormones, and the like will ensure the continuity of the entire organism.

The cell membrane carries out two seemingly opposing functions. It must keep wanted things in and unwanted things out. At the same time, it must also allow outside wanted things in and push out inner unwanted things. For instance, every cell needs to discard the waste products of its own metabolism, diffusing them across the membrane from which they will be taken away by the bloodstream. If the cell fails in that task, it will die of self-poisoning. It also needs to sponge up outside oxygen, glucose, and other goodies for use as cellular fuel; otherwise it will die of starvation. For these reasons the cell membrane is identified as semipermeable, and that semipermeability makes exchange across the boundary both possible and necessary.

Our body's most fundamental building block, the cell, holds one of our most powerful contemplative metaphors: semipermeability. We could also call it *selective permeability*. Our essential nature is built upon a physical foundation of give-and-take, discernment, exchange. We can't afford to be either impermeable or boundaryless. A more lyrical way to put it is that a cell possesses neither a separate sense of self nor selflessness. We hold ourselves together, and then we let go of self—in a discerning way—into a relationship with what is around us. By holding ourselves together, we can do work that contributes to the sustainability of the whole organism. By exchanging ourselves with the outside, we also contribute to our well-being.

Biologists use the metaphor of breathing to explain this process. They call it cellular respiration: taking in needed resources and releasing what is no longer needed. Buddhist teachers such as Thich Nhat Hanh call this *interbeing*. Each cell in the body *inter-is* with all other cells and the fluids they swim in. Cellular semipermeability may function as a template for our understanding of relationships, of interdependence and interrelatedness. We may assume that these concepts come from the capacities of our mind to grasp the nature of existence, but these principles are realized on a moment-to-moment basis, in a very practical way, in our physical form. By becoming more bodyful, we can begin to experience our interbeing on a more immediately useful level.

Taking In and Letting Out Practice

Take a comfortable position, standing, sitting, or lying down. Take a few minutes to check in with your body, listening to sensations and allowing yourself to just experience them. See if there are any small or simple movements that would feel right for your body as it is now. When you are ready, say the phrase "taking in" to yourself a few times, and just notice what happens in your body. What images, sounds, memories, and emotions arise when you say these words? What history do you have with this phrase? Right now, how are you experiencing your body taking in air, light, and sound? Then say "letting out" to yourself a few times. Particularly notice how your body responds to these words and what associations you have to them.

When you feel ready, repeat this process with the phrases "keeping out," "keeping in," and any other metaphor for permeability (or a disturbance of it) that comes up for you. End the exercise by checking back in with your body for sensations and respond to them with small, simple motions. You may want to write down, briefly and descriptively, some of the experiences and associations you had.

Tissues

In our bodies, clumps of cells and the fluids around them—collectively called the matrix—specialize in ways that cause them to hang out together, like with like, working more efficiently as a group, like a family. When this happens, they can perform dedicated functions, and they earn the name *tissue*.

There are four basic types of tissue in the body: epithelial, connective, muscular, and nervous. Epithelial tissue covers body surfaces (think skin), lines inner body cavities, and forms glands that secrete oil, sweat, enzymes, and hormones. Connective tissue, the most abundant tissue in the body, binds organs together and protects and supports the body (think bone, fascia, ligament, and tendon). Muscle tissue (such as heart, gut, and biceps) contracts and stretches to make movement possible. Nervous tissue initiates and transmits electrochemical impulses that coordinate body activities (think nerves) into a symphony of effective actions.

When we study the tissues of the human body, we can begin by listing the impressive number of actions that tissues undertake. They cover, line, secrete, bind, filter, protect, support, move, and coordinate. When their function is to secrete something, they are called glands (think thyroid or sweat). Together, all these glandular actions help the body maintain *homeostasis*. Homeostasis relates to our need to be in balance at a fundamental level, hovering around predetermined, optimal set points. The human body "wants" to have a temperature of 98.6 degrees Fahrenheit. Our blood wants to have an acid/alkalinity balance (pH factor) right around 7.40 (7.0 is pH neutral, like water). Our blood sugar normally sits at 90 milligrams per 100 milliliters. We need a precise ratio between oxygen and carbon dioxide in our body, a moment-to-moment negotiation that depends on our arousal and level of activity. The main biological definition of stress is something that upsets our internal homeostasis, something that causes our temperature to rise, our blood sugar to fall, and the like. The tissues of our body are constantly operating so that stressors don't overwhelm biological equanimity and make us sick. They work to establish and maintain homeostasis. Homeostasis, in this sense, may be our mechanism for experiencing imperturbability and our moment-to-moment and metaphoric equanimity.

One thing that science has recently come to appreciate is that the word *homeostasis* may be a misnomer. The word derives from *homeo* (the same) and *stasis* (standing still). Our tissues are not still but rather in a constant state of active engagement, oscillating back and forth between ranges, even if those ranges are very small, similar to the slight balancing corrections our body makes while standing on one leg. In fact, researchers are now beginning to think that health can be seen as a function of how adept the body's tissues are at constantly and actively shifting to maintain balance—oscillating back and forth, if you will. For instance, medical researchers now look to heart rate variability—the capacity of the beating heart to sensitively speed up and slow down to changing circumstances—as perhaps the most powerful indicator of heart health. It's not that we want to avoid going out of balance (because that is how we change) but that we want to be adept at coming back into balance. This brings up a contemplative teaching popularized by the psychotherapist Sheldon Kopp. In his classic book *Back to One*, he tells a story of young monks being taught a meditation technique that involves counting—one, two, three, four . . .—until their mind interrupts with a thought and they have to start over again at one. Several of the monks boast to each other that they can get all the way to twelve, or even twenty. A quiet monk in the back shakes his head and notes that he rarely gets above four and that he always has to go back to one. Unbeknownst to the group, the teacher has been listening, and he comes over to the quiet monk, puts his hand on his shoulder, and announces that it's the monk who can go *back to one* repeatedly who deeply understands the practice. Going back to one metabolically is a bit like coming home; both leaving it and coming back have their merits.

Health, from the sense of tissues in the body, isn't so much about stillness but rather an almost athletic ability to stand on one metabolic leg. More importantly, it involves the ability to return to that stance over and over, on shifting ground. With this acknowledgment, people are now using the term *allostasis*, which centers on the idea that we can maintain stability through the process of change. Here again we experience change and oscillations as foundational to our understanding of bodyfulness.

How much change is healthy, and how much is too much? Our body is constantly negotiating how much to change in the service of balance. What researchers are beginning to discover is that some stress, called eustress, is crucial to our health because it exercises the tissues, keeping them active and strong, much like physical exercise is crucial for muscle development and health. But stress that is too great or, even worse, too prolonged—called distress—causes trouble.

Change is fundamental for health, but it comes at a price, especially if it's too sudden, intense, or chronic. However, evidence is mounting that if we are physically comfortable most of the time, our tissues are not exercised enough and can lose capacity to bring us back to balance. Balance in this sense involves challenging ourselves by using modest daily stressors to exercise our tissues and optimize cellular potency as well as seeking to minimize stress that can't be used in that way.

Literally and metaphorically, our body and our being are built to exercise our capacity to change constantly in small ways so that when large change is demanded of us, we are ready for it. We will build upon this concept of engaging in a little in order to be able to cope with a lot in the next sections of this chapter.

Research shows us that contemplation, sitting meditation, or moving meditation can provide a kind of vaccination against too much stress. We will see in subsequent chapters how challenging bodyfulness practices, such as sensory awareness, coupled with attention to breath and conscious movement, can challenge us, prevent the loading on of distress, and help us recover more quickly from destabilizing stress.

Before we leave the level of the body's tissues, one more physiological process bears our scrutiny: inflammation. Inflammation occurs when the body senses the presence of some kind of injury or pathogen. Inflammation protects, defends, and returns us to allostasis by making sure that toxins or bacteria in a certain area are contained locally so that immune cells can more easily neutralize them and so they don't spread throughout the body. It does this by causing blood vessels at the site of an injury to dilate and leak out cells that kill bacteria and help heal the wound. This action can produce heat, redness, swelling, and sometimes pain. The swelling keeps the injury or pathogen isolated to as small an area as possible.

The strategy of isolating an injury, both to heal it and keep it from spreading, echoes throughout our body and behavior. Psychologists have long known, for instance, that we tend to "wall off" threatening emotions and push fearful or inconsistent thoughts and memories into the unconscious. If we consistently experience an emotion as toxic and try to wall it off, our body reacts much like having an autoimmune disease—we are attacking ourselves, constantly attacking an emotion as if it were a toxin.

In psychotherapy, this chronic compartmentalization goes by the name *defensiveness*, where we react fearfully and aggressively when our old walled-off hurts are activated. Contemplatives often call this our ego, and it can definitely get inflamed. If we don't find the resources to deal with the patterns established by the original injury, the feelings and thoughts remain isolated, swollen, and suffering. The task of psychotherapy and contemplative practice is to reduce this inflammation, to gently and bravely examine old wounds by relaxing the ego/inflammation in a safe environment. Isolating a perceived toxin can be temporarily useful as well as painful. If this action is chronic, so is the inflammation. Chronic inflammation is now thought to be at the root of many, if not most conditions and diseases, such as autoimmune disorders, allergies, some heart disease, and even some cancers. It may be that the metaphor of chronic inflammation holds true for thoughts and feelings as well as body tissues. Our bodyfulness project is to consciously track sensations, breathe, move, and relate to others in ways that make the emotions and thoughts usable for our return to balance. As we progress through the chapters of this book, we will return again to this process and study how to increase our resources for healing through the vehicle of bodyfulness.

Balancing Practice

Let's experiment and have a bit of fun. If you can stand comfortably, stand. Start by rocking your weight, oscillating front to back, side to side, and up onto your toes and back down. Notice when certain places in the oscillations may be challenging to your balance. Let the natural asymmetry of your body be there—no need to make the left side wrong for destabilizing more quickly than the right, for instance. If possible, let the oscillations be playful; let catching yourself before you fall be as fun as possible.

If you want to keep experimenting, play with standing on one leg for a bit. Just like the monks counting one, two, three, four . . . , the aim isn't to stand on one leg for a long time so much as it's about noticing your body as it begins again to lift up one leg. What muscles seem to activate to allow you to stand on one leg? What happens when you focus your awareness on these muscles, supporting them with your attention? What images, memories, sounds, or feelings come up when you play with your balance? Change to the other leg and notice the small or large differences between the two. One leg is being the stable one, while the other is being mobile. Stability and mobility are crucial body metaphors you can work with. When you are done with your one-legged standing, you may want to write down a few words or images that come to you when you attend to the words *balance*, *stability*, and *mobility*.

Organs

Just as groups of cells band together to form tissues, groups of different tissues aggregate to take on a definite shape and form, and perform a specific function. When they do this, they are called *organs*. The skin, for instance, isn't only a tissue but also our biggest organ; it holds within it hair, nails, nerves, veins and arteries, fat tissue, oil glands, epidermis, dermis, and elastic fibers. The skin performs many functions and, like all organs, is essential for our survival. It helps control our body temperature; protects the underlying tissue from bumps, bacteria, harmful light rays, and from drying out; and stores and synthesizes crucial compounds such as vitamin D. Our brain is also considered an organ and can be thought of as a huge nexus (a center of connectedness) for the nervous system. In general, the rest of our organs hang out in our torso, examples being the heart, liver, lungs, and stomach. As a bodyfulness project, consider studying the locations and functions of the different organs (appendix A).

Organs—aggregations of different cells, tissues, and glands that live and practice together—might be seen metaphorically as local communities, much like sanghas, churches, temples, or mosques. This level of organization occurs because the body needs more complex, whole-body, somatic processes—such as digesting, breathing, or pumping blood—that use both slower circulating fluids and quicker electromagnetic pulses to communicate. Our organ-based contemplative metaphor relates to the body's need to gather and coordinate resources from farther and farther afield, and to trust in the special knowledge and skills of other specialized structures. Such need requires that we develop a diverse and complex community identity. Later on we will look at organs again and see what they can teach us about community; about how to work and practice together for a common purpose.

Systems

Our last level of organization before we become a whole organism is the system. As you might imagine, a system is an association of organs that have a common function. Our systems are the digestive, nervous, muscular, skeletal, endocrine (think all kinds of different secreting glands such as pituitary, pancreas, and thyroid), cardiovascular, lymphatic, integumentary (the skin is also a system), respiratory, urinary, and reproductive. Appendix B lists the workings of each of the body's systems.

At the level of the body's systems, we can begin to work with overarching bodyfulness principles more clearly. The first principle, oscillation, may be how the body's physiology creates a blueprint for our concept of the middle path. In humans, the body systems tend to oscillate between expansion and contraction. The heart pumps: blood gushes in when it expands, blood is sent on its way when it contracts. Muscles contract and stretch. The lungs expand with air, then deflate to release that air. Our stomach and intestines expand and contract (peristalsis) to process food into nutrients and eliminate waste. Some organs squeeze out chemicals that regulate our homeostasis. As we noted before, our brain waves are a kind of oscillation, a back-and-forth modulation of electromagnetism that functions much like a symphony conductor.

Systems in the body may echo the function of systems in societies. As complexity continues to develop, another layer of specialized and far-flung coordination evolves. That coordination takes the form of diverse oscillations.

Basically, the body systems pulsate in a synchronized way, all the way from the cellular to the systems level. Life contracts and expands along a continuum, and that continuum has two endpoints (extremes) and a middle. We move between the two extremes of expansion and contraction, and we spend the most time somewhere in the middle. This is where the famous bell-curve shape comes from that we see on so many graphs—it describes the state of being in the extremes occurring under rare conditions and increasing amounts of time passed in the center of some capacity or state. The middle tends to feel normal, like being in between, in neutral, or at rest. Health in the body sense isn't so much about stopping and hanging out in the middle as it is swinging through it regularly. The middle path is just that—a path we walk along, swinging our arms and legs back and forth, back and forth.

The themes of stability and mobility enter again on the systems level, when we look at the skeletal system. In part, our bones function as levers that move via the contraction and stretching of the muscles attached to them. In order to have multiple levers that can generate all kinds of different movements, we have joints. Some of these joints help us be stabler, such as the elbow and knee. Called hinge joints, the elbow and knee can only move in one direction— back and forth, like hinges. This allows them to help carry weight and keep us vertical. Other joints generate mobility, most notably the ball-and-socket joints at the shoulders and hips; they permit movement in all three dimensions. Interestingly, we tend to see stabler joints alternate with more mobile joints: in the arm, the shoulder is more mobile, the elbow is stabler, the wrist is more mobile, and the knuckles are hinges. The same occurs in the leg. Metaphorically, we operate best when we can oscillate along a continuum from very stable to very mobile; from finding center and grounding there, to leaning forward and taking off in new directions.

We can easily make the mistake of thinking the body's systems are separate, doing their own thing as individuals. As we saw at every other level of body organization, this view may be convenient but it's wrong. In fact, most of the body's systems link together in such an interdependent way that they can't function even momentarily without each other. Some liaisons are stronger than others. The nervous system, for instance, which uses sensations to understand how to coordinate activity, hooks up so intimately with the muscle system to produce movement that biologists term it the *neuromuscular system.* Whether it's a speeding up of the contractions of the heart muscle or the shortening of some skeletal muscles so that we lean into our friend's touch, sensory nerves are always going to hook up with muscles that produce responsive actions. And those actions generate more sensations, and the loop strengthens. Bodyfulness specializes in working with this sensorimotor loop. It promotes sensory awareness as a way to strengthen the loop, which becomes disrupted in conditions of trauma and stress. It also supports conscious movement responses that help restore a sense that our actions in the world are effective and satisfying. More on this in chapter 6.

Another powerful alliance knits together the nervous system with the endocrine and immune systems. Feedback loops between brain chemistry, hormones and enzymes from the glands, and cells in the immune system create constant cellular conversations that zip throughout the whole body via multiple circulation routes. These conversations always carry information that helps systems assess risk, current state, demands on the body, appraisals of what is going on outside the body, and the like, such as how the digestive and immune systems turn off in response to endocrine signals of stress.

We also organize a close partnership between our viscera (our gut organs and systems) and the emotional centers of our central nervous system. Neuroscientists call this our *viscerolimbic loop*, which is a fancy phrase used to validate "gut feelings." Basically we form many of our emotions, before we are even aware of them, from a back-and-forth feedback loop between our midbrain and viscera. When our metabolism changes, due to changing circumstances, such that our adrenal glands start secreting stress hormones, for instance, the middle and center parts of our brain coordinate a behavioral response by forming an emotional state of fear. The emotion of fear helps direct our actions in reaction to whatever is perceived as fearful. The adrenaline-based fear response in turn instructs other gut systems to turn off so that more energy can be mobilized for self-defense. This is likely where the knot in our belly comes from.

Interdependence

Psychoneuroimmunology is a relatively new field in behavioral medicine that specializes in understanding these powerful liaisons between systems. More rightly it should be called psychoneuro-*endo*immunology, as the endocrine system is also intimately involved. This research field basically investigates the influence of emotions, beliefs, and other cognitive and psychological states on immune function, nervous system sensitivity, and stress levels, and vice versa. The bottom line of its findings: how you think and feel matters greatly to your health. Physical and mental/emotional health *inter-are* in the body's systems and therefore in the whole body itself.

Another area of inquiry in behavioral medicine finds that the vagus nerve, which is a nerve with branches running from the heart, lungs, and gut, also strongly connects to the muscles of the face, jaw, and voice box. It's thought that parts of this nerve play a central role in social engagement, or using direct communication with another to help us calm others or ourselves in order to understand each other and resolve conflicts. Professor Stephen Porges is credited with developing the polyvagal theory that makes these connections between nerves and behaviors.

The vagus nerve has three divisions, the first of which moves our eyes, ears, facial muscles, and voice, allowing us to use speech (style and tone), listening, and contactful looks to engage with and work things out with others. By practicing with and athleticizing this upper division of the vagus nerve, called the ventral vagal complex, we may begin to more consciously practice nonviolence in our relationships.

Research notes that if we can't use social engagement to work things out with someone with whom we are in conflict, then the second vagal division kicks in. This middle branch of the vagus nerve, embedded within the sympathetic nervous system, activates our fight-flight defenses by speeding up our heart rate, priming our lungs with more air, and secreting stress hormones that make us anxious and put us on high alert. In this state of activation of the body, our reality becomes one of self-defense. We run, cower, yell, or hit. These actions are more primitive and more metabolically stressful than social engagement. However, on rare occasions one or more of these actions may be the only strategies that work to get us out of danger.

The third and lowest division of the vagus nerve, the dorsal vagal complex, is where we go when all hope of relational repair or self-defense seems lost. This branch of the nerve turns down life functions to such a low level that we may be in danger of our heart stopping. It may be the mammalian equivalent of playing dead, as it produces a fainting response, a collapse, a kind of catatonic and dissociative calm.

Psychologists think the lower vagus may also be involved in the concept of *learned helplessness*. (Do an Internet search on this term. The story of its discovery and development is a fascinating and macabre tale.) This theoretical concept states that if we are repeatedly exposed to situations of suffering where nothing we can do will relieve our suffering, we will eventually learn to just give up. We will, in essence, begin to believe that we are fundamentally helpless to do anything about our circumstances and become passive to them, even in the face of evidence that we can indeed help ourselves. We become habituated to helplessness. Living through child abuse, growing up in poverty, war, and oppression will do this.

Contemplative practice may over time provide those of us who suffer from learned helplessness with novel experiences of increased control over our internal state, most notably mental and emotional ones associated with the vagus nerve in the gut and the emotional centers in the brain. We can confront learned helplessness by challenging our habitual ways of interpreting our experiences and by practicing activism at its most basic level—by moving purposely to get something done. This might start simply by challenging ourselves to keep working a bit longer on untangling a knot or sticking with a difficult interaction until we feel understood. What may be equally if not more effective is for us to find bodyfulness practices that strengthen the ventral vagal complex, the part of us that can oscillate between speaking and listening, and between broadcasting and receiving emotional states. By working directly with the body, perhaps by learning to breathe more deeply, to move more responsively, and to open our mouth to talk things through, we can directly alter our experience so that we are not chronically creating suffering we assume we can't avoid or have to be defensive about. In the face of suffering that we can't change, we can also reach out to others for help as well as ally with others as a means of generating stronger and more effective activism.

Movement Continuums

As our last look from the systems level of body organization, we can say that the various systems of the body work together to provide us with continuity or continuousness. When respiration, digestion, circulation, and metabolism all coordinate, we operate harmoniously along a series of continuums. When we dance for a few minutes in the living room, our skeletal, circulatory, respiratory, and muscular systems work together to produce a continuum of movement.

Observable movement starts at the primitive level of reflexes. As we jump and turn, automatic reflexes that contract muscles to keep us from falling over or unbalancing kick in. Primitive motor plans learned when we were young children help us jump, clap, alternate our left and right legs, and reach out for our dance partner. More complex dance moves learned as preteens show up and entertain us as we execute the twist, a moonwalk, or a one-two-three waltz step. At the creative end of this movement continuum we spontaneously invent moves that delightfully express the synergy of the music, the moment, our mood, our smiling dance partner, and our efforts to avoid bumping into the coffee table.

Movement, as we noted before, is so fundamental to life that its absence defines death. It operates along a continuum from highly automatic to highly spontaneous and creative. The body echoes various continuums, most of which may express our phylogenetic evolution from single-celled organisms to multisystem creatures. As well, these continuums reflect our personal developmental journey from a single-celled fertilized egg to the grown-up reading this book. The continuum begins with automatic and inherited operations that occur below and outside consciousness and will. It ends with highly creative and highly conscious actions.

Martha Eddy, a well-known movement educator, has developed practices called *somatic movement* and *mindful movement*, which may be related to these ideas.[1] She notes that by practicing conscious sensing and conscious moving within a contemplative framework, the moving body can be an entry point to activism. This is because working from a base of conscious movement allows us to directly experience our motivations for acting as well as increase our ability to modulate our energy, skills that any effective activist can use. We will look more deeply into these ideas later in the book.

What the body shows us, via simple observation, is that the primitive workings of the body don't go away and aren't wrong. They keep operating throughout our lives, forming an infrastructure that our more complex, systemic operations rely on for support. We are both primitive and complex; otherwise no spontaneous dancing in the living room is possible. It doesn't work to make our more automatic selves "less than" our more "evolved" conscious selves. They are not separate. They exist on an interdependent continuum that expresses both a personal and collective continuity, a unity of all life. That is bodyfulness.

By studying the structure and the function of the body on both literal and metaphoric levels, we can formulate a guide for practice. In this way we can examine handed-down somatic disciplines and decide whether or not they still work for us. Or we can adapt them via our emerging and ongoing authoritative knowledge of the body. We can also use the practice suggestions below as a way to make up our own ways to address our needs and interests as we experiment with our relationship to bodyfulness.

Chapter Practices

- This bodyful contemplation involves lying on the floor if you can. Begin by checking in with your body, as well as playing with small, simple movement adjustments. When you feel ready, begin to play with expanding and contracting your body. You may oscillate between spreading out as far as you can, arms and legs wide and extended, then, at whatever pace feels right to you, curling up your body into a kind of fetal position. Feel all the muscles and bones that have to work together to produce these movements. Experiment with this back-and-forth a few times, noticing various sensations, images, memories, or other associations that arise. Does expanding your body feel scary or delicious? Does making it smaller and curled in feel comforting or confining? There are no right or wrong associations; just notice. What metaphors arise that might be useful to work with?

- The three branches of the vagal nerve (aka Porges polyvagal theory), discussed above, carry useful metaphors for how we deal with conflict in relationships. Take a few minutes, perhaps with a pen and paper, to reflect on these three strategies:

1. The first strategy is to talk it out and stay connected with someone via eye contact and a calm and connected voice tone. It involves an ability to listen as well as speak.

2. The second strategy is to ramp up and defend yourself by getting angry and aggressive or to flee and retreat.

3. The third way is to power down, to lose energy and motivation; to get sleepy or distracted; or to feel numb, depressed, and helpless.

Take a moment to attend to each of these three strategies, perhaps remembering a time when you used them. Which of these strategies do you tend to use the most? The least? Do you tend to use a certain strategy with a certain person, according to gender, age, or position of power? One strategy isn't better than the other; we need to match them to differing situations. However, the fight-flight and the faint strategies are more expensive and stressful to the body than the staying-connected strategy. You may want to jot down a few notes about each one, either memories, habits, or body costs. Then put the pen down and attend separately to instances of each of these three strategies. Attend to your bodily sensations and impulses to move as you bring each one to your attention. Hold these bodily reactions in your awareness, holding them with your attention as if you were holding a small child.

- Let's go back to the living room and get a feeling for the dance continuum discussed early in the chapter. First, put on some music that makes you want to move. Then, if you can, just stand there with your feet together, feeling the contact of your feet with the floor. Now let go a bit in the muscles at the front of your ankles. This will likely make you start to fall forward. As you start to fall, notice when the "righting reflex" kicks in: muscles on the back sides of your ankles, legs, back, and neck will contract to straighten you up as you automatically take a step forward to catch your fall. All complex movement is built on reflexes such as these, working together primarily to keep you safe.

Now let's try some simple motor plans. You practiced these endlessly as you learned to sit up, crawl, and walk. They are second nature now. Just play with them consciously, as a part of enjoying the music. Some of the most common ones are reaching, pushing, grasping, and pulling. Notice how easily they become familiar gestures, perhaps with personal significance. Pushing can develop from learning to push your hand against the floor in order to stand up from sitting; later it can become "Stop!" when you want to signal someone to stay back. Reaching can feel like "Come to me!" Grasping might bring up memories of holding something and saying "Mine!" These ancient motor plans seem to correspond to basic psychological states, likely developing together evolutionarily.

Now bring in those dance moves that you secretly or not so secretly practiced as a kid. Whether you perfected your Lindy Hop or your hip-hop, take some time to have fun with your cultural and social past. Dance moves such as these help us identify as a member of a group as well as just have some fun. We have to learn them from scratch, but reflexes and motor plans help us put them together in a (hopefully) artful way.

Lastly, let the music move you "freely." No learned moves come into play; just let yourself do whatever seems to show up. It doesn't have to look like any dance you ever learned—in fact, it works best when it looks like *no* dance you've ever learned. This kind of movement gets compromised when we try to think our way through it ("What do I do now?") or if it dredges up emotions of embarrassment or self-consciousness ("I must look like an idiot."). As much as possible, just label those critiques as thoughts and feelings, and go back to the direct experience of moving your body freely.

How did that feel? This was a conscious movement practice, a short experience of developing bodyfulness by experiencing a continuum of movement. We will complexify it as we go along.

- To explore the body systems (cardiovascular, muscular, digestive, and so on), the respiratory system is often a good one to start with because it's so accessible to our awareness. Find a comfortable position, either standing, sitting, or lying down. Take a few minutes to rest your attention on your breathing. Notice any tiny movements or sensations that seem to come from that system—for example, the rising and falling of your chest or abdomen or subtle sensations around the nostrils. See if you can notice across your body a range of subtle to more gross movements that accompany your breathing. If you are feeling a bit playful, see if you can slightly magnify the tiny movements you notice. Take these few minutes to "be with" your respiratory system, perhaps noting some of the things it does ongoingly and how it interacts with other systems.

- You can try this with other systems too. For instance, you can feel your pulse and track your heartbeat. You can alternate tensing and relaxing different muscle groups. You can indirectly feel your nervous system by attending to the physical details of how calm or excited you are, details such as a racing heart, a jittery feeling, or a relaxed exhale and loose muscles.

- In your digestive system you can pay close attention to the acts of drinking or eating, noticing the details of the transition of food or water from the outside to your insides. In this same system you can pay attention to your stomach once the food or water lands there. Being able to accurately sense the fullness of your stomach before it's strongly distended by a big meal correlates with good eating habits. You can also feel your lower intestines and colon contract and release (peristalsis) as you get ready to go to the bathroom. Being able to cooperate with your digestive tube's natural processes makes for a happy digestive system.

PART TWO

Bodyfulness Practice

Presencing Bodyfulness

3

———

Sensing

THE POET WILLIAM Blake once wrote that the body would be the soul's prison if the five senses weren't fully developed and fully opened to the world. He stated that it wasn't just the eyes that were the "windows of the soul" but all five of the senses. Common wisdom holds that we possess five senses: vision, hearing, touch, taste, and smell. Anatomical accuracy tells a slightly different story.

Kinds of Sensing

It can be argued that we also have a sixth sense, but it's *not* intuition. Intuition surely occurs, but it's most probably related to our ability to use *any* of our senses in subtler ways. For instance, we may intuit that a friend is angry, even when they haven't said anything about it, because we are paying good, strong, and open attention to the extremely subtle changes in the muscles of their face, whether we realize it consciously or not. We are reading their micromovements that are almost always involved in a person's experience of their emotions (whether they are consciously aware of the emotions or not). While intuition can be error prone, this sensing of subtle actions and states in oneself and others forms the basis of a good psychotherapist's skills as well as those of an attuned parent or a lover. It's likely involved in our feeling more deeply understood by some people over others; they are literally paying more attention to the smaller and quieter signals our body gives off and responding sensitively to those signals. Intuition certainly assists us with our authoritative knowledge of our body. Bodyfulness builds this overarching sensory skill. We will come back to this idea of subtle sensing a bit later.

The true sixth sense—true because there are specialized sensory neurons in the body for it—is kinesthesia, our awareness of the position and movements of our body.[1] Kinesthesia-based sensory neurons are linked with the types of muscles that attach to our bones and then contract to create movement through space or to hold our position in space.[2] Think kicking with your leg. In order for kicking to occur, your muscles need feedback from sensations that tell you where your leg is in the first place (under the torso, to the side), whether or not you have weight on it, whether it's bent or straight, and how much muscle contraction is already going on. All this needs to be taken into account before you can even begin to organize a good kick. Other examples using the same process include curling your fingers, sitting upright without support, or walking across the room.

Kinesthesia tells us where we are in space, which muscles are contracting, and how our body is oriented in that space. The sensory neurons associated with kinesthesia are embedded in and around our joints, and within the muscles themselves. We will work more with kinesthesia in the movement chapter, but for now it's enough to know that we operate with all these senses in order to provide the central nervous system with data about what is going on inside and outside of us, data that is used to organize responsive actions.

Kinesthesia Practice

One of the best ways to challenge and develop kinesthesia is to play with a young child. If possible, get down on the floor with one and roll, wrestle, somersault, nudge, and hold. Handicap yourself so that you can play like this on equal terms. This kind of stimulation is crucial for child development, but it can also be a wonderful bodyfulness project for you. If you don't have young kids in your life, some other options are swinging on a swing set, playing with a dog, or taking classes such as aikido or modern dance. It's also fine to roll around on the living room floor with another adult!

When we think we have six senses, we still are ignoring our *interoceptors*, the sensations going on deep inside the body that monitor our metabolism and our arousal. Am I thirsty, cold, hungry, or in pain? Do I feel the pleasant tingle of sexual arousal? Is my heart beating fast? The insides of the body move around, in their own way, so they need to know how much to move and when. Inner sensation is critical for the body's ability to take care of itself. The vagus nerve we talked about in chapter 2 is a good example of a sensory nerve that monitors our inner goings-on. Besides helping us monitor our inner well-being, interoceptors have been correlated to emotional intelligence and the ability to make good decisions: the more we can track our inner state, the more we literally know what we feel; and the more we know what we feel, the more we can know what we want as well as understand the feelings of others. Can we call this a seventh sense? Anatomically, it makes sense (so to speak . . .). A chart that organizes the various senses we have just talked about can be found in appendix C.

Gut Feeling Practice

"Gut" feelings often shape and guide our emotions. In emotional situations, as much as possible, pay attention to your inner sensations—in your belly, chest, and the contraction of your muscles. Don't search for an emotional label for the sensation. If a label arises naturally, that is fine, but just take it under advisement rather than getting attached to it as an explanation. Just let yourself experience the emotion as a physical event and notice how the emotion wants to move you. Does it want to make your hand into a fist? Does it make you smile? Does feeling it give you shivers? The more you can surface these connections between feeling, sensing, and moving, the more nimble and bodyful you become with your emotions.

What the Senses Monitor

If we want to look at our seven senses further, we can group them according to what they are monitoring. We have senses that monitor the external world, often called exteroceptors. Our vision and hearing form this group. We have senses that monitor our borders, such as taste—we are sensing something that was outside but is coming inside via the mouth—and smell, as we sniff molecules in the air that enter our nose. Touch that is sensitive to pressure can be in this group, as it senses something making contact with our skin. We could also put kinesthesia in this group, as it tracks our body's relationship to the space around it. Lastly, we have senses that arise in the interior body, our interoceptors. Our body, in order to survive and thrive, needs to monitor the external environment, our borders, and our insides. Our bodyfulness practices will keep all of these in mind, both literally and figuratively. This might be a bit different than other somatic disciplines, which tend to favor attending to the body's internal sensations (often called body awareness). While inner sensing is crucial, bodyfulness values all types of sensory processing and advocates for a cooperative balance between the different types of sensation.

In fact, favoring one sensory mode over another might be involved in mental and emotional instability. Keeping our attention outside of us for too long can be equated with hypervigilant monitoring of other people and things, leading to anxiety and false attributions. Keeping our attention at our borders for too long can lead to excessive worry about what is coming into and out of our body. Excessive internal focus has been shown to be a marker for hypochondriasis, body obsession, and overblown worry about minor sensations. Balance and attention that is free to both focus and oscillate is key to well-being, so that one type of sensation can provide a check and balance to the others.

Inside, Borders, and Outside Sensation Practice

Let's take a minute to experience the types of sensation. First, close your eyes and pay attention to inner sensations. Start by just noticing, and then move toward purposefully putting your attention to different areas inside your body, such as your heart beating, lungs expanding and releasing, body temperature, sensations of pain and pleasure. Next, open your eyes and look around as well as listen to the sounds around you. Just enjoy the looking and listening outside of you for a moment, taking in the physical details of the objects and the space around you.

Then turn your attention to the position of your body. Notice the sensations of knowing whether or not your knee is flexed or extended, which parts of your body are vertical or horizontal, which parts are touching the furniture or the ground. You might want to change your position so you can feel the difference between them. Lastly, become aware of your skin, noting the feeling of clothing against it and the places of pressure where your body rests against the support of the floor or the furniture. You may want to touch your arm or some other part of your body both lightly and with pressure. Play for a bit with changing into different positions and noticing how sensations change as a result. Which type of sensation seems easier or more familiar? More or less interesting?

How Sensitive?

We have been looking at what and how we need to sense. Now let's look at how much or how little we need to sense. Not surprisingly, the wisdom of sensory input seems to follow a middle path, as we get into trouble either with too little or too much of it. Human senses are only able to pick up a small percentage of the spectrum of data out there in the world. Take vision, for instance. Light comes in many forms, depending on its wavelength. However, our eyes are constructed to only pick up visible light. No infrared or ultraviolet light for us, unless we're assisted by elaborate machines that can pick up these waves for us. We simply don't have sense organs that can pick up everything that is out there, which can be humbling. We all know that dogs can hear better than we can, and sharks can smell much better than we can. Due to energy conservation, life-forms evolve sensory organs that are specialized to pick up data related to that organism's needs and interests, and no more. What our senses pick up is what we think is real, yet reality is relative and different for different organisms.

In fact, one of the most important functions of the nervous system is to *eliminate* information so that we can further optimize our limited data-gathering energies. We do this through a series of sensory filters located throughout the nervous system. These filters strain out sensations according to the principle of energy conservation: since my conscious awareness is expensive, what is the most important sensation to pay attention to right now? Our sensory filters constantly shuffle sensations between the foreground of our awareness and the background, where they can be ignored or processed subconsciously. We have some control over some of these filters via neuroplasticity (that is, what we practice). An example of having good sensory filter control might be the ability to tune out background noise in a coffeehouse as you attentively listen to a friend's voice. Our ability to oscillate our attention between different sensory foregrounds and backgrounds in a disciplined way forms one of the central bodyfulness skills that we will practice. In a way, we are athletically toning our sensory filters and becoming sensory athletes as a result.

As we know, too much sensory input can be overwhelming and destabilizing, even for a sensory athlete. We have all experienced sensory overload and wanted to get out of a noisy restaurant or a crowded market. Sensory overload has been routinely used as a form of torture (blaring music, being kept awake). Attention deficit disorder (ADD) and its relative, attention deficit hyperactivity disorder (ADHD), and perhaps autism, are thought to be based at least partly in problems with the central nervous system's processing of sensation. The sensory filters are not working properly and the person becomes easily overwhelmed by too much sensory input and can't make sense out of it—that is, determine what is truly important—by foregrounding and backgrounding.[3] Imagine what it would be like if you couldn't put the sound of your friend's voice in the foreground and all the sounds in the room came at your ears with equal weight. It would all be chaotic noise and very stressful.

Sensory deprivation can be equally harmful. Too little sensory input can also be a form of torture, as in the examples of solitary confinement and early childhood neglect. Sensory-rich environments—ones that contain different, interesting types of stimulation—have been shown to enhance emotional and cognitive intelligence and problem-solving as well as contribute to resiliency. Sensory deprivation can also be played with productively, as when we quiet our inner and outer environments during meditation. Extreme sensory deprivation needs to be temporary, however. Research using sensory deprivation tanks shows that when deprived of sensory stimulation too long (multiple hours), most subjects start to hallucinate and dysregulate.

Again, a balance between differing amounts of sensory input can be key to well-being. As on any middle path, most of our time is spent with moderate and varying amounts of sensory input, yet we remain capable of short periods of intense stimulation as well as hardly any. We can use quiet moments to recover from a hectic day and have fun at a noisy and chaotic family reunion. We can engage with sensations without overly identifying with them, a core contemplative practice. By balancing the types and amounts of sensory stimuli, sensation can be experienced as one of our body's ongoing and ever-changing "senses" of self that we can greet, deeply relate to, and then let go of as the moment passes. Bodyfulness involves a purposeful and athletic ability to alter our attentional focus so that the amount and type of sensations we work with can be nourishing and deeply informative.

Sensing, Awareness, and Attention

Working with the senses presupposes that we are attending to them consciously. For instance, in order to see properly, we need to focus the lens of our eye using tiny muscles around the eyeball. This kind of active focusing occurs in all seven of our senses, so much so that we can understand sensing as an active, engaged process that involves muscular effort in many cases. This concept can help us understand the differences between awareness and attention. Awareness forms a kind background state of consciousness where largely automatic, body-based oscillations occur that monitor our inner and outer situation. Attention is even more active, requiring more conscious (and often muscular) effort. We always attend *to* something by focusing our conscious awareness, pulling certain stimuli from the background into the foreground. When we're attentive to certain sensations, we actively draw them into the foreground where they can be experienced in a heightened state of consciousness.

High-quality attention sits mostly in our middle path, in the bell of the bell curve, oscillating according to different circumstances. If we can't focus our attention enough, we feel dull, sleepy, distracted, and inept. These states often coincide with an overall low tone in the body. If our attention is dialed up too strongly, we tend to experience tunnel vision, hypervigilance, and anxiety. These feelings often go hand in hand with excessive tone in the body. In either place—very high or very low tone—our ability to work with sensation and with our situation can be compromised.

We need to go to these extremes in specific situations, such as letting go of attention in order to fall asleep or riveting our attention toward a source of danger. But most of our day, hopefully, falls in the middle ground.

Meditation of any kind trains our ability to pay high-quality attention. Working to gain control of our attentional muscles parallels athletic training. The result, in the case of bodyfulness training, is more developed, nuanced, and acute sensing, along with the ability to focus and unfocus attention at will. We practice, we increase our attentional tone, and we become attentional athletes. From a meditation perspective, we could even say that monks and nuns are Olympic attentional athletes. Bodyfulness practice takes this metaphor quite seriously; it sees the training of literal muscles as related to the training of attentional muscles. We will work with this idea more in the coming chapters.

Chapter Practices

- Next time you are sitting down to an unhurried meal, take some time to notice the smells and tastes of the food as it enters your body. These are moments where your senses of taste and smell are saying yes (or perhaps no) to something that was outside of you and different from you that will now come into you and in many ways become you. What associations and metaphors occur to you as you put the food into your mouth, chew it, and swallow it? *Savoring* is the word we often use for this sensory experience.

- Take some time throughout the day to notice what type of sensory mode you use more than others and when. For instance, if you work in front of a computer for a living, you are using your eyes a lot. If you are a construction worker, you, more than most people, are reading your body's position in space and its muscle contractions. Does this ever feel like overuse? How do you recover from a day spent mostly paying attention outside yourself? Or an extended time being very internal? Do you notice that you weren't using one type of sense much at all? What kinds of activities might be fun for you to experiment with that would provide a different and more balanced sensory palette across your day?

- This practice is based on the Focusing technique developed by Eugene T. Gendlin. Begin by setting the space: private, quiet, and undisturbed. Now, as before, begin by taking a few moments to check in with your body, making sure to attend to each part with as much detail as feels helpful. Then ask yourself, "What wants my awareness right now?" It could be a body sensation or an issue you are dealing with that registers in your body in some way. Make contact with that body state or issue. Describe it to yourself and attend to your body as you do so. Acknowledge what comes up in your body, and tell it you are listening to it and working to be with it. See if it's okay to just be with it in a state of curiosity. Listen to it from its point of view. Does it have its own emotion or mood? Let it know you hear it and see if there is anything more it wants to tell you. Then let it know that it's time to stop, but that you will be back soon to listen again. Thank your body for speaking about this issue. Afterward, just let the experience of focusing on yourself keep working within you. Don't try to analyze or categorize it. Just trust that this deep listening will work in the background to provide support and inspiration as you go back into your day.

- The next time you are with a friend or family member, pay special attention to them as they speak to you, especially about something important to them or emotional for them. Really take in the small details of the look on their face, their voice tone, their posture and gestures, and the speed at which they speak and move. Try not to analyze what you are taking in but rather let yourself form impressions that guide you to respond in ways that show that you are listening not just to their words but also to how they feel.

4

Breathing

CONSCIOUS BREATHING PRACTICES have been used as a healing strategy for longer than we can know. These practices have been
seen by many, throughout time, as a kind of royal road to physical, emotional, psychological, and spiritual health and well-being.
Bodyfulness walks this royal road. The Latin root of the word for
breath, *spir*, as with the words *inspiration* and *expiration*, corre-
sponds to the word *spirit*. Many traditions feel that breath and spirit
are one. Yet today there are so many conscious breathing practices
out there—some of which even contradict each other—that it can
get overwhelming. In spite of this, conscious breathing persists as a
powerful, self-organized, relatively simple, and amazingly effective
means for leading a bodyful life. The efficacy of this practice lies
in the fact that we are breathing already, about twelve times a minute, every minute of every day, until our very last minute of life.

To begin our understanding of the power of conscious breathing, we need to distinguish between our normal everyday breathing habits and breathing practices we do temporarily in order
to generate certain effects. Rapid panting, for instance, is used in
some yogic traditions and birthing techniques as a way to cleanse,

manage pain, or increase energy. No one advocates for doing this day in and day out. Ultimately you will decide what specialized and temporary breathing practices, if any, are best for you, under conditions that work for you. What this chapter will do is help you to assess what breathing practices are best for you. The main emphasis will be on your moment-to-moment process of breathing with and through everyday experiences. In other words, we will seek to develop good, basic breathing habits that largely operate in the background as we attend to other things.

Physiological research has weighed in on this issue. The physical benefits of everyday good breathing have been well and thoroughly documented. They can be summarized as improving immune function; regulating arousal; decreasing sinus problems; balancing hormones, enzymes, and neurotransmitters; stabilizing blood gases; increasing vitality; promoting digestion, circulation, and proper organ function; facilitating waste metabolism; aligning posture; decreasing muscle tension; and increasing motility and mobility. These physical effects can in turn be seen as having a profound influence on psychological well-being, particularly in the areas of mood, the reduction of negative emotion and increase of positive emotion, emotional regulation, and the capacity for social engagement. But what does good breathing look like?

Generally, "good breathing" involves three elements: (1) the balance of inhale and exhale, (2) an easy and mobile flow through the body, and (3) an ability to adapt quickly and effectively to changing internal and external events. These three characteristics of good breathing trace their origins to the physiology of the respiratory system.

Let's start with the balance of inhale and exhale. Here we can go back to the concept of biological set points that we explored earlier. At all times, it's critically important that our blood gases, most notably the ratio of oxygen and carbon dioxide, are balanced in our body. The ratio can alter slightly and briefly in response to changing circumstances, but basically this isn't a set point you want to mess with. If these two gases get out of balance, our pH balance alters and we become too acidic or too alkaline. In dramatic cases, such as with scuba divers and the Apollo 13 astronauts,[1] this imbalance can quickly kill you. However, a slight imbalance can also be chronic, often a result of a habit of overinhaling or overexhaling. A chronic imbalance between inhaling and exhaling likely contributes to many diseases and adverse health conditions, both physical and psychological. If we don't balance our inhale to our exhale, we get sick. In balance, our breath can be one of our greatest means of healthful living.

Next, breath needs to flow in and out easily, with a minimum of fuss. At rest, an inhale actually involves effort, mostly the contraction of the diaphragm muscle, a domelike sheath that cradles the underside of our lungs. When the diaphragm muscle contracts, its dome flattens out, passively urging our lungs to expand and allowing air to whoosh in. During exercise or intense experiences, the respiratory system recruits other muscles to inhale more deeply (between the ribs, around the neck). Our exhale, on the other hand, is an act of letting go. For most of the air to leave the lungs, we release our muscles and let gravity do the work. Gravity is really good at things like this. Only during exercise or intense experiences do we need to actively push out the air. This back-and-forth oscillation brings in new oxygen from the atmosphere because we use oxygen as fuel for all cellular activities. As a product of these cellular activities, the body generates excess carbon dioxide, which builds up and must be exhaled. We need both oxygen and carbon dioxide in order to function, so the contraction and release of muscular effort, both at rest and during more intense experiences, can either facilitate or inhibit the efficiency of this process. As any person with asthma or panic attacks can tell you, how intensely we contract and let go, plus the timing of this alternation, predicts distress or well-being.

Our last good breathing characteristic involves the ability to alter our breathing in relationship to changing events. This simply means that we can access more oxygen when we need to or off-gas more carbon dioxide if we need to, given the demands of the moment. Can we inhale more deeply as we run down a path? Can we let go, relax, and exhale fully when it's time to go to sleep?

Stress, certain diseases, and even different psychological issues are often associated with certain breathing patterns that are so locked in that we can't change them when circumstances change. For example, we might have habituated to not breathing deeply enough, causing a difficult situation to feel worse or a pleasurable situation (such as sexual pleasure) to be dampened. When our breathing is in tune with our internal state and our external environment, we navigate life more bodyfully.

Although the relationship of good breathing to physical health seems obvious, its relationship to psychological health might be less visible but no less important. Many theorists and clinicians agree, for instance, that breathing is affected by conscious and unconscious attempts to stave off strong emotion or uncomfortable states. Researchers also believe that we dampen our perceptual sensing when we restrict our breathing, which results in feelings of anxiety, fear, or numbness.

Neuroscientists have found that the brain's primary emotional center, the limbic system, plays an important role in breathing patterns. Respiratory functions exist throughout our limbic system, our olfactory area, and our language centers, linking breathing to our emotions, sensations, and speech. Researchers have found that rapid or shallow breathing can *induce* emotions of anxiety and fear. This creates a negative spiral that can itself induce further anxiety, panic, and negative interpretations of what may be occurring. How we breathe correlates to how we cope. The good news is that positive emotions, specifically laughter, affect our breathing and our subsequent coping in positive ways.

We begin to learn breathing patterns in the womb, as we listen to and rock with our mother's respiration. This learning process continues as we are held against our caretaker's chest, sensing directly from their breathing rhythms whether we are safe or unsafe, calm or excited, erratic or stable. We directly internalize the breathing patterns of the people around us, wordlessly and without conscious attention. As we grow up and reach adulthood, with practice we can choose how to breathe for ourselves, according to who and where we are now. This conscious choosing of our breath, our spirit, opens the door to a bodyful life. Choosing to be a conscious breather involves both specialized and ongoing efforts.

The relationship of breathing, sensing, and emoting is critical not only to emotional "fluency" but also cognitive intelligence. Poor breathing habits and unbalanced breathing can decrease our ability to sense our emotional states and act on them appropriately. Good breathing habits facilitate emotional stability and positive feelings. Because of this, breathing can be a powerful agent in creating both physical and psychological regulation or dysregulation. In bodyfulness practices, we understand that physical and psychological states occur interdependently, and conscious breathing therefore forms a central role in our practice.

Specialized Breathing Practices

A number of current contemplative and psychotherapeutic traditions maintain that specific breath practices can help alleviate symptoms of illness (mental, emotional, and physical) through raising body energy levels, increasing the breath's adaptability, and activating the body's natural flow. The techniques used to accomplish this, however, may be in some contention. Some classic body-centered psychotherapists believe that deep, rapid breathing through an open mouth can help overcome our emotional defensiveness by cathartically breaking through defenses to deeply buried feelings. This technique is also said to heighten sensation for those who feel numb or out of touch.

This idea of using increased breath volume and rate to liberate emotions and increase energy contrasts with views held by other psychotherapists who work with the body. Many now believe that the practice of deep rapid breathing can be dangerous, can induce psychological distress and crisis, and likely can precipitate anxiety attacks due to hyperventilation. Instead, some therapists and clinicians suggest that we must *reveal* the *natural* breath through attention and patience, gently coaxing it out of hiding. Trying to alter breathing through mechanical, forced exercises may have little effect on our breathing habits themselves because these temporary methods don't change the fundamental patterns that have taken time to develop. Rather, we practice so that the breath happens freely, during moments of conscious attention. Tantric and yogic traditions abound with very specific and detailed breathing practices, some of which might be more arousing and cathartic, and some more calming and restorative.

Taken together, all these traditions seem to home in on two

general strategies: one advocates for conscious breathing that energizes, activates, and breaks through psychological blocks; one calms, allows, and releases. Both strategies value mobilization and vitality, though they might define those terms differently. On the surface, they seem contrasting and even contradictory. But these two paradigms also sound a lot like our breath itself: the slightly arousing physiology of the inhale and the relaxing and letting-go physiology of the exhale. Perhaps we can use both these types of practices in a bodyful manner, choosing each according to our own bodily knowing.

How to Choose a Specific Breath Practice

Specific, freestanding breathing practices can be a useful part of our bodyfulness tool kit. However, what works for some of us may not work for others, and our own changing needs will lead us to choose different practices at different moments. For instance, sometimes we will use a breath practice for physical health, sometimes for emotional stability, and sometimes for spiritual exploration. Different purposes lead us to different breathing practices, though during any practice it's important to breathe in ways that support our ability to track sensations and feel both stable and mobile.

In order to choose wisely, led by your knowledge of the body and its principles, you can follow a few sensible guidelines that help you with breath practices handed down from various traditions, or you can modify them or make up your own:

- *Know your breath patterns.* Observe your breathing in both calm and stressed states. This means that you describe rather than analyze or judge your breathing, simply noting whether it's slow or fast, deep or shallow, more in your belly or more in your chest, and so forth. Your assessment can include the following aspects: the three-dimensionality of your breath; the flow of movement through various body parts (especially the torso); the balance of the inhale to the exhale; your patterns of effort as you breathe; your respiratory rate; how your breath relates to your emotions and arousal states, checking to see if your breath may be supporting or interfering with that state. Basically get to know your breath during challenging as well as normal circumstances. Does the breath practice you are deciding upon support this self-knowing?

- *Cooperate with natural oscillations.* Breath oscillates. Getting in alignment with this biological truth may help you reestablish healthy breathing and learn to use your breathing as a means of regulating other body oscillations, such as those in the digestive, cardiovascular, endocrine, and nervous systems. Experientially, this feels like a cooperative back-and-forth between the inhale and exhale. This doesn't mean that the inhale and exhale are in a fifty-fifty lockstep—often the exhale takes more time than the inhale, for instance. But they should feel connected and mutually supportive. This kind of physical balance likely predicts emotional and psychological balance as well. Does the breath practice you are choosing help you feel this cooperative back-and-forth?

- *Teach yourself to regulate yourself.* You will likely benefit from learning conscious breathing practices that stabilize and repattern your breath habits and that can be called upon outside the learning environment and during stressful moments in daily life.

Can these breath practices be used anytime or anywhere, when needed? Being able to practice good breathing throughout the day goes a long way toward our self-directed dissolving of dysfunctional breathing patterns over time. As well, it empowers us to self-regulate rather than depend on instruction. Does the breathing practice you are considering help you with this?

- *Breathe in relationship.* Breathing is catching. How you breathe influences how others breathe around you, creating a kind of breath community. In this sense, you want to become a good breather as a resource from which your family, friends, and co-workers can benefit, as this modeling effect can exert its own healing momentum in the social systems you occupy. Does the breathing practice you are choosing help you with this?

- *Learn to breathe with feelings.* Since emotion and breath coregulate each other, you can use conscious breathing as a resource during emotional moments. It's important to engage with how you *really* feel, more than *how much* or *how little* you can feel. In this way the breath practice can be used to support your emotional processing rather than exaggerate it to levels that are unwarranted, inauthentic, or not advisable. Does the breathing practice you are considering help you with this?

- *Use breath practice as a resource for both up- and down-regulation.* You can learn conscious breathing practices that are both activating and calming, and you can use them both, much like your inhale and exhale naturally occur together. In this way you re-create the organic oscillations of your healthy body. Does the breathing practice you are considering help you with this?

- *Allow time for conscious respiratory change.* Be patient with your breathing patterns. Because breathing is mostly regulated by the autonomic nervous system, it takes time as well as practice to change long-standing breathing imprints. Sustainable changes in ingrained breath patterns can take months of conscious practice to generate increased balance in ongoing breathing. It may be powerful or exciting to do a breath practice in a class or a retreat, but does that practice help you breathe differently on an ongoing basis? Does the breathing practice you are thinking about taking up acknowledge this?

The Balanced Breath Practice

Given the above guidelines that can help us intelligently choose special breathing practices, how can we use them to help facilitate each breath as it moves us from moment to moment? How can we become a better breather at the bus stop, in a meeting, in our lover's arms, or when we hold our children? I would like to offer what I call a balanced breath practice.[2] By learning it you can practice it on your own, first in more neutral states and then under stress. You can easily invoke the practice when you need to regulate your state or assist someone else's. Practice it in the sequence below for a minute or two or for extended periods of time. It works best to practice it in different positions (such as sitting, standing, lying down) as well as while moving. Practice it when it feels useful and easily done. One of the best times to practice it is when you are just waking up or when you are about to fall asleep, as your nervous system is a bit more pliant at these moments. Ultimately the practice becomes the habit of good breathing. You will learn this practice in short chunks so that it's easy, but as soon as possible you will want to put the chunks to-gether into a seamless whole.

- Start with just the inhale. Just let your exhale take care of it-self while you attend to your "inspiration." The inhale, as we learned before, takes effort. The task of this phase of breath-ing is to make the muscular contractions as efficient as possi-ble, neither under- nor overworking. In order to facilitate the easiest contraction of the diaphragm, you will do what might be called belly breathing. This involves allowing your breath to be felt all the way down into the floor of your pelvis. You are obviously not inhaling the air anywhere but into the lungs, but by mobilizing your belly via the metaphor of breathing down into it, the dome of the diaphragm can flatten more eas-ily, which passively expands the lungs so that they draw in air easily. This also avoids the upper chest breathing pattern that is associated with unregulated emotion and anxiety. Take a moment to practice the inhale, as if each one makes your belly a bit more rounded and full; as if you can feel your inhale all the way down into the bowl of your pelvis. Do this first with a larger breath, so you can really feel it, and then try it with a more normal volume of breathing. Remember, it's not about how much air you can take in each time; it's not necessarily about "more air is better." It's about how easily and gracefully you do the work of inhaling, which occurs naturally when you relax and mobilize your belly. Take as much time as you like to play with inhaling such that your belly moves with you, while other parts of your body relax and support that action. Play with the inhale in different positions. What metaphors emerge when you focus on your inhale? Is it okay to make this small effort without struggling or working too hard? Can effort be easy? Use this practice to uncover buried associations you may have to what it means to make constant small efforts to affirm your aliveness through the inhaling breath.

- Now for the exhale. As we noted before, exhaling while at rest is an act of letting go. Some of us may associate letting go with collapse, helplessness, or a loss of control, making the exhale a scary thing. So it can be important to use this part of the practice to consciously cultivate the distinction between actively cooperating with gravity and passively and helplessly giving up. The direct experience may feel as if each individual rib is resting closer together on the exhale,[3] and your weight is being supported by the chair or floor. Really feel the weight of your torso as you exhale. Over time, this can give your body a direct experience that it's safe to rest and that gravity can be helpful. Take some time now to focus on the exhale; just let your inhale take care of itself. Play with the exhale in a variety of positions. Focus on the release of effort as a way to accomplish the exhale. As you let go on the exhale, can you let go a bit more at the end? If you are sitting up with no back support (recommended), all the big muscles in your back, shoulders, and chest can release, leaving just the tiny, short muscles that attach one vertebra of your spine to the next to efficiently hold you up. Each exhale can be an affirmation that some things can be accomplished by letting go of effort.

- Now put the inhale and exhale together as an integrated practice, alternating between pooching out your belly slightly and then releasing into a feeling of your weight being supported by the ground. Just practicing the efficient activation of the inhale and the pleasant release of the exhale can be enough for many of us. At first you can practice this as a stand-alone exercise (in order to get the hang of it), and over time you can invoke it as a way to make your current state accessible, manageable, and productive.

- If you would like, you can learn the advanced practice of balanced breathing, which involves working with the transitional moments between inhaling and exhaling. To begin, work with the transition from the inhale to the exhale. Restricted inhaling often squeezes the torso into a narrowed and elevated shape, making you feel that your breath is going straight up and down. "Rounding out" the transition from inhale to exhale can help keep your body three-dimensionally flowing with the breath wave. It may be useful to imagine that at the top of your inhale there is a rounded shape, so that the inhale can "roll over" easily into the exhale rather than be pushed over.

- The next advanced practice is to work with the end of the exhale. When we experience ourselves as calm and safe, we tend to pause naturally and ever so slightly at the end of the exhale, where our body waits to be "inspired" to inhale again. The advanced exhale practice takes advantage of this and simply allows this natural pause to emerge on its own. It's important not to force it to happen, as this defeats the physiological pause and disrupts the relaxation of the cycle. Simply watch for and greet the pause if it shows up, and bear witness as your body organizes itself to inhale again on its own physiological authority. In both of the advanced practices, notice what associations emerge from them, as any conscious breathing will bring up potentially powerful and useful contemplations.

- If you are ready, put all four practices together—inhale, roll over, exhale, pause. Enjoy!

The above balanced breathing practice represents a possible play project in the development of bodyfulness. It's important to remember that our breath, like our fingerprints (and for that matter, our whole body), is unique. You know best how you breathe best. Trust your own experiments with breathing, and trust your judgment regarding the use of both handed-down practices and those of your own invention.

The Purposes of Breath Practice

Conscious breathing practices follow different purposes, as we noted above, and knowing what purpose you are currently serving can augment your work with breath. Below are four models for what we might want to accomplish with breathwork practice: a relational model, an energy model, a regulation model, and a consciousness model. All four models use the balanced breath practice as a starting point and tailor more challenging practices from there. These models can be used interchangeably, according to your needs and goals.

RELATIONAL MODEL

Breathing is a social and communal process as well as an individual one. Beginning in the womb and persisting throughout our life span, our breathing patterns are influenced by what others are doing. As we noted before, in early development infants' autonomic nervous system "listens" to the breath patterns of those around them and harmonizes their patterns to those of their caregivers, habituating to others' breath signatures. In adult relationships, one's breathing is continuously affected by the quality of interaction with others, whether it be calm, stressful, sexually aroused, happy, or fearful. Nonverbal communication research, for example, notes that when people who like each other interact, they tend to breathe at the same rate, and they tend to hold their breath or sigh at the same moments, creating a respiratory *pas de deux*.

Therapists often note that in order to stay in relationship with someone, it's best if you breathe and oscillate your contactfulness (such as looking at and away from one another) at the same time. This might be difficult when the relationship is uncomfortable or conflictual. Often breathing becomes tied up in defensive strategies that break connection and relationship. Perhaps one person in an interactional system who is breathing in a way that supports calm engagement could influence others in the system to do so as well. It may be that you can experiment with the role of being a good breather as a relational and "respirational" repair strategy. In this way you use your own regulated breathing as a direct intervention in the service of healthy relating.

Breathing Together Practice

Find a friend or companion who is willing to breathe with you in this exercise. Sit next to each other (shoulder to shoulder) and each take a minute to check in with your breathing as it is. No need to change it. Now, still sitting next to one another, each of you rests your hand on the middle of the other's back so that you can feel the movement of your partner's breathing. First, the person on the left will play with changing their breathing to match their partner's, just for a minute or two. Notice what changes in you as you breathe together with your partner. It may be a very different or very similar pattern. How does it feel to accommodate their way of breathing? How does it feel to breathe similarly? Now switch roles, with the person on the right syncing their breathing to their companion. What do you notice? Lastly, just breathe the way you breathe while at the same time noticing differences and similarities with your partner's breath. The aim here isn't to breathe like other people but to notice what associations come up when you are in close contact with others' breathing. Likely these associations have something to do with your models for how relationships work.

ENERGY MODEL

Psychotherapists, physicians, and contemplatives maintain that conscious breathing can increase available energy and vitality in the body. The energy model uses conscious breathing to reestablish waves or pulsations of fluids, gases, and tissues in the body that support a natural state of aliveness. In this model, breathing practices can generate more "energy," though the term *energy* has often been loosely and vaguely defined. This model is often associated with feeling and expressing emotions, though not always. Many people make the common error that for maximum well-being, energy always has to be "raised." What we now know about bodyfulness shows us that we actually want to feel that we can both raise and lower our energy levels in a nuanced dance with internal and external happenings. Conscious breathing that sensitively modulates our energy as well as accurate emotional expression can be resources for unblocking physical and psychological tensions, and allowing a flow of natural and pleasurable experience.

Two Energy Practices

If you are up for it, find a space where you can move around. It might be best to be standing for this one if you can. Begin the exercise by taking some deep, full in-breaths, down into your belly. Let your exhales out by letting go into gravity. Do this for a bit, no more than a minute, and stop doing it if you feel some kind of symptom, such as pain or dizziness. After getting more air in this way, or as you stop the bigger breaths, just move around freely, having fun with it, so that your muscle contractions can use up the extra oxygen you have inhaled. This exercise is designed to help you gradually learn to tolerate the extra energy you get by breathing more, in a friendly way. It could be that you can only take a breath or two before you need to move around. That is fine, more isn't better. The whole exercise should not take more than a few minutes. Again, more isn't better. It's about gradually finding new set points for your energy. To be safe, it might be best to postpone doing this exercise if you suffer from any respiratory or cardiovascular diseases. (This exercise is adapted from Gay and Kathlyn Hendricks's Radiance Breathwork system.)

The next exercise should be done while lying in bed, preferably just before going to sleep. Again, be your best judge as to whether or not this exercise works for you. It simply involves emphasizing your exhale a bit more as you fall asleep. Exhaling fully tends to be calming, though the calming effect only occurs if your exhale is just slightly fuller than your inhale. The important feature of the practice is to let go into gravity on the exhale, feeling your weight sink into the bed. This letting go can apply to various muscles as well; just feel the weight of various parts of your body resting into the bed as you exhale.

You can do the reverse in the morning, just before you rise from bed. Take a few moments to emphasize your inhale slightly. You might find that this energizes you as you start your day. Both these practices can be used in the middle of your day if you need to calm down or ramp up. All in all, you want to be able to work with your energy levels in a friendly way, and your inhales and exhales present an excellent means of achieving that.

REGULATION MODEL

Conscious breathing can regulate our physiological state as well as our emotional and psychological states. Breathing is intimately tied up in the physical regulation of our metabolism; we can feel this directly every time we breathe in a way that calms us down or revs us up. As we have seen before, our metabolism needs to constantly adapt to changing conditions. Emotions are themselves a temporary change in our metabolic rate. From a biological standpoint, emotions are designed to come and go as a way to form adaptive responses to the internal and external environment. Trouble arises when they don't come (repression or suppression), they don't go (overidentification), or they become mismatched to the current situation. In these instances, emotional and psychological dysregulation occurs.

The regulation model of breathwork practice uses conscious breathing to help us stay within tolerable parameters on emotional and physiological levels, and be neither too aroused nor too depressed to be able to function. In this model, our breath works to support a state in which we are able to pay good attention to our current state and to stay mobilized and empowered within it.

Breath Regulation Practice

In relationship to the regulation model, we want to adapt the previous breath exercises to situations in daily life where we feel challenged by something and need to adapt our energy to meet the challenge.

The next time you are in a mildly challenging situation, take a moment to discreetly alter your breathing so that it helps you meet the challenge. This might mean emphasizing your inhale or exhale a bit more. Or it might mean doing the balanced breath practice. The idea is to recruit your conscious breathing to regulate your state. Think of this practice as the first thing you do, even before you try to solve the challenge. The practice readies you to meet the challenge more effectively.

CONSCIOUSNESS MODEL

Many ancient languages such as Latin, Greek, Gothic, and Arabic use words for *soul* or *spirit* that are related to the ideas of breath, air, or wind. In Greek, for instance, *psyche* or *pneuma* is synonymous with *breath*, *soul*, *air*, and *spirit*. In Latin, the term is *anima spiritus*, meaning "breath" or "soul." *Ki*, in Japanese, means "air" or "spirit," and in Sanskrit, *prana* connotes a resonant life force. In Chinese, the character for *breath* (*hsi*) comprises three characters that together mean "of the conscious self or heart."

Throughout the ages, conscious breathing has been seen as eliciting mindfulness, expanded awareness, raised consciousness, and spiritual connection. In many cases, this breathing involves slowing down and paying close attention to the details of the inhale and exhale. Breathwork can also be linked to transpersonal states in which we feel connected to others, to all life, and to all that is. We can employ different yogic and tantric breathing practices to clear and center the mind and heart. In many cases we use them to enhance connection to a more unified sense of self and the world. In the consciousness model, set practices tend to dominate, though different ones promote different goals, such as meditative states, cleansing, energizing. A common denominator is the search for a clear mind and body so that higher states of consciousness may emerge.

Consciousness Breath Practice

Did you know that when ten of us are in a room, chances are that one of us is breathing in a molecule of air that Einstein had in his lungs at some point in his life? How cool is that! We are all connected. We all exchange molecules with one another. We also engage in exchanges with other life-forms, most notably plants. Did you know that trees breathe in carbon dioxide and exhale oxygen? This demonstrates interbeing at a highly pragmatic and literal level.

Take a few minutes, in any position that feels right for you, to do a breathing meditation. Start by focusing on the exquisite detail of your breath, just as it is. Then, if it feels right, as you stay with your breathing, begin to reflect on associations to breath that feel meaningful to you. It might involve your interrelatedness with trees, your connection to others, or your sense of the divine. With each breath you can touch this connection, this interbeing. It's both inside you and outside you. Breath enacts your semipermeability, your fundamental oscillations, and your spirit.

Conscious breathing practices call upon many traditions and serve many purposes. By knowing which purpose we want to work on, and by having a strong sense of our historic and current breathing patterns and the associated states that accompany them, we can breathe our way to more bodyful states. We start with a balanced breathing practice that constitutes home base. From there, we can experiment with specific exercises that inform and challenge our old ways of breathing as well as lay down new habits that increase our vitality, our ability to stay connected to others, and our work toward more awakened states.

5

Moving

As we noted before, movement defines life, and working consciously with our bodily movement taps into our aliveness and our bodyfulness in fundamental ways. Movement of any kind involves doing something that changes our position, location, or state. Movement is how we take any kind of action. Because of this, movement carries physical, psychological, and contemplative possibilities. Physically, the structures of the sensorimotor loop—sensations firing up nerve pathways that morph into responsive actions, which in turn stimulate new sensations—can guide us in understanding our inner and outer world with a new level of clarity.

Our body moves in many different ways, for different purposes. We need to protect ourselves. From knee-jerk reflexes that help us avoid falling when we stumble to motor plans that coordinate our running away from danger, we move to preserve our bodily integrity. We also preserve ourselves by accessing needed resources, such as food and water, which usually involves locomotion, that is, moving from here to there. We move to communicate, as when we wink, wave our hand, vibrate our vocal cords in speech, or point our finger. Similarly, we move to relate to others, by leaning against them in moments of closeness, for instance. And we move to express our creative impulses every time we dance or sing. Because movement accomplishes so many different things, different types of movement have evolved.

MOVEMENT CONTINUUM					
METABOLIC	TONE	REFLEXES	MOTOR PLANS	NVC	CREATIVE
↓	↓	↓	↓	↓	↓
Cellular	Freeze	Simple	Reach	Voice Tone	Play
Tissue	Faint	to	Push	Touch	Sponta-
Gland/		Complex	Grasp	Posture	neous
Organ			Pull	Gesture	
			Yield	Gaze	
			Walk		

Automatic _____ Semivoluntary _____ Voluntary

Constrained _____ Unconstrained

Less Conscious _____ More Conscious

Metabolic Movement

To understand the many types of movement we make, we can create a continuum. Beginning on the left of the chart, we see the movements we share with many other life-forms, motions we do automatically, without conscious direction or will. These movements tend to be small and come to us prepackaged via our genetic inheritance. They often involve pulsations of some kind, such as the wavelike expansion and contraction of cells, tissues, and organs, in ways that don't use skeletal muscles. While we can't control these movements directly, we can influence many of them indirectly. When our heart beats fast during stressful events, we can pause, breathe slowly and deeply, and work to calm ourselves. This often slowly decreases our heart rate because we are altering the physical triggers we *can* control that cause our heart to beat faster. Often these movements can't be observed directly either. Because they are small, often internal, and largely done automatically, they remain mostly private, personal, and harder to track by ourselves, let alone by others. Because these movements occur automatically, nature conserves energy by not setting up many interoceptive sensory neurons to track them.

Psychologically, these small, usually quiet pulsations may be a kind of physical unconscious, on par with Freud's idea of the psychological unconscious. Our automatic actions form the bedrock of our existence, our identity even, yet remain largely in the shadows. Bodyfulness involves journeying into this physical unconscious, illuminating what can be seen, much like Freud did with the psychological unconscious. These movements may also help us identify with other humans, animals, and other life-forms because all life patterns itself on these basic actions. As human beings, we have the opportunity to cultivate a more sensitive and friendlier relationship to many of these buried movements and increase, to a certain extent, our ability to work with them more directly. We could say that this generates a more awakened and bodyful state.

Automatic Movements Practice

Create some quiet and undisturbed time. Find a comfortable position that is easy to sustain. Turn your gaze inward, and focus your attention on any small, repeating movements happening in your body—your heartbeat, for instance. For most of us, it's hard to track our heartbeat unless it's really pounding hard. Just take your time, and refrain from putting too much effort into it. Just listen for it, and don't worry if the signal is faint. If you want, you can put your fingers to your carotid artery in your neck or to the pulse in your wrist as an aid. Alternate feeling your heartbeat under your fingers and just listening without the aid. When you feel ready, use your hand or your finger to tap out your best guess as to the lub-dub of your heart. Notice how this feels, to be doing your heartbeat in your hand, consciously. Do any thoughts, images, or feelings come up? Practice this as often as you like. The more you recruit voluntary muscles, such as those in your hand, to replicate involuntary movement such as your heartbeat, the more you may gradually increase your ability to track and work with it.

To extend this practice, slow your tapping slightly and see if this slows your heart (this works in conjunction with relaxing and breathing slowly). Try it for speeding up the heart slightly as well. Remember, the tapping is only a suggestion. The heart operates from an ancient intelligence and almost always knows best how frequently to beat. Trust your heart.

To extend the practice a bit more, try this exercise in more challenging circumstances, such as at your desk at work or when you are feeling emotional. This may help you over time to respond more sensitively to these challenges via your increased ability to consciously participate with and trust your physical state of being.

Another more psychological variation is to listen to your heartbeat as it is and imagine that it's talking to you. Could there be a simple message in the lub-dub? Like "All is well, all is well" or "Pay attention, pay attention"? Try not to impose a nifty phrase on your heartbeat. Instead, let your attention get a bit dreamy and just see what floats up into your awareness. This exercise is designed to thin out the barrier between the conscious and unconscious parts of yourself, much like any good psychotherapy will do, in order to access buried resources in the form of images, feelings, and symbols. It doesn't work when you think too hard. (Thinking hard often thickens the barrier between the conscious and unconscious parts of ourselves.) If you get a sense of the heart message, take some time to be with it, relate to it directly, hold it in your attention carefully and compassionately.

TONE

When we begin to involve skeletal muscles in the production of movement, our first actions on the continuum are small, largely automatic, and only partly under our control. They have to do with the nature of muscle cells, which are long and fibrous. These muscle fibers are wrapped together in bundles to form individual muscles. When they contract, they get shorter, and this shortening pulls on our bones to create movement through space. When these fibers are completely slack, we are said to be in a *hypotonic* state, which works well for resting, falling alseep, and letting go in general. When they contract, the fibers shorten maximally, and we are said to be in a *hypertonic* state. This state works for moving around, lifting and carrying, and all kinds of work in general. In the middle ground lies the state of tone, where the muscle fibers are contracting just enough to take up the slack but not enough to produce a motion. This state specializes in being alert, ready, and attentive.

Some of our most primitive defenses involve body tone. Fainting (or playing dead in some species) involves extreme hypotone. Freezing in place involves hypertone, often involving equal, simultaneous contractions of opposite muscles (such as a flexor and an extensor) so that tension but no overt movement ensues. The young of many species will employ freezing or fainting as a way to deal with danger, and some species, such as the deer in your headlights, use it throughout their lives. Defensive hypertone often involves two other classic defenses: fighting and fleeing. Because these defenses involve motor plans and practice, they tend to be used more by mature members of a species. Often psychotherapists working with trauma survivors will notice disturbances in their clients' body tone, where survivors get caught up in repeating hypertoned or hypotoned defensive actions. Helping survivors find the broad middle ground of bodily tone, where they feel calm but alert, heralds recovery.

Body Tone Practice

Take a few minutes to experiment with your body tone, while standing, sitting, and lying down. First find the extremes by trying to let go as much as you can without falling, just letting yourself slump, collapse, and feel your weight against the floor. Notice what happens to your attention, emotions, and associations. Then work with tensing up in ways that don't produce much if any observable movement. Notice the associations and feelings here. Then find your middle ground, where you feel your muscles are primed but not pulling on your bones. This can take a bit of practice, and some parts of your body may be more practiced at it already. Notice how it feels to be in this calm, alert place. What associations do you notice with this state?

REFLEXES

Our next type of involuntary movement shows up in our reflexes. Reflexes use muscles and help keep us safe and sound as well as form the platform for more complex and voluntary motions. They are so important that purposefully stimulating them constitutes one of the primary ways we evaluate newborns for their developmental well-being. Reflexes start simply, hooking up one sensory nerve, such as the one at our kneecap, with a motor neuron in a muscle, in this case the quadriceps on the front of the thigh, bypassing the need to recruit the brain to take the time to figure out what action to do next. In case of emergency, such as a stumble, the sensory neuron enters the spinal cord and connects directly to a motor neuron, which causes the muscle to contract quickly, which extends our leg (called the knee-jerk reflex) and hopefully keeps us vertical. Reflexes start to get more complex when they group different muscles together in a coordinated action, such as the orienting reflex. This reflex turns our body toward a sudden sound or other startling stimulus and often involves twisting our torso, turning our head, and lifting up our arms. Complex reflexes coordinate themselves in the brain through practice.

Reflexes have the reputation of being quick but dumb. We can startle at benign things, or the reflex can be so strong that it unbalances us even more than the original event. In prolonged psychological trauma, reflexes can become either hyperactive, causing us to jump at the least little thing, or hypoactive, where they don't activate when they should. Being a newborn and an infant is all about getting increasingly sophisticated reflexes to come online and to balance one to the other (such as flexing reflexes that are just as strong as extending reflexes in particular parts of the body). When our reflexes work well, we then make use of them to coordinate whole actions, such as crawling and walking. We all know that gaining this bodily knowledge in the early months and years of development helps infants feel secure in the world. Building on reflexes during physical play and investigation of the world forms an essential part of this process.

Reflexes Practice

Bodyfulness practices that work with reflexes follow similar pathways as previous exercises, where motions that are automatic are practiced more slowly and deliberately. Reflexes tend to curl up or straighten out a part of the body or the whole body. They can also twist the body. If you are willing and able, clear a space on the floor and lie down. After checking in with sensations for a bit, begin to slowly flex and extend fingers, toes, wrists, ankles, knees, elbows, shoulders, and hips, in any order. Just have fun with it, eventually seeing if you can combine these movements so that you might roll over or twist. Make sure to include your spine. Notice how it feels to do this. Let it be as experimental and playful as possible. This is how you did it as an infant. You might notice, for instance, that an extension of your arm can become a reach and a curling of your arm can become a grasp and pull. Playing like this can be very recuperative for a body that has spent the day in an office chair or driver's seat. It can lessen stress and fatigue as well as improve your mood. This is because moving your body in ways that purposefully parallel reflexes can be like coming back home.

Semivoluntary Movement

Now let's look at semivoluntary movement, typified by our breathing. Our lungs are wired with both automatic and voluntary nerves, such that we can ignore our breathing and it will go on just fine or we can pay attention to it and consciously alter it in some pretty fundamental ways. Because of this, every major spiritual tradition as well as virtually all somatic practices use conscious breathing to influence our current state as well as our long-term breathing patterns. We began the practice of consciously working with breath in chapter 4, so in this chapter we will focus on the movement possibilities inherent in purposeful breathing.

Breath Movement Practice

As before, find an undisturbed time, place, and position. Begin by checking in with sensations. Now turn your attention to your breathing, which is an easily observable semivoluntary movement. Much like in the previous chapter's exercises, take time to simply observe and be with your breathing as it is; try not to judge it or change it. When you feel ready, use your hand to gently replicate the rhythm of your breathing, letting it rise and fall in the air or go back and forth in time with your breathing. By replicating the motion consciously, you can learn over time to feel it more. If you are feeling a bit adventurous, deliberately put this breathing wave into other parts of your body, such as your whole arm, your feet, and your legs. At some point you may want to play with your whole body purposefully moving with the rhythms of your breathing. What associations come up with this breathing movement? For some, it brings oceanic images, as the waves of breath rise and fall. Notice the expansion and contraction your body tends to replicate. What images or feelings rise up when you expand? When you contract? Expansion and contraction are fundamental oscillations, used frequently by the body as the base upon which more complex movements are organized. They tend to carry psychological associations as well. Does it feel a little risky to get bigger? Does getting smaller bring up memories? Does one oscillation feel like work and the other one like letting go? Is it hard to work or hard to let go? By working with both the physical and psychological aspects of movement together, you can use one to support and inform the other in creating a more bodyful state.

MOTOR PLANS

The body holds other interesting semiprogrammed movements we can play with. Evolution has noticed there are certain basic human movements we use so often that it makes sense to genetically preprogram a strong motivation to practice and perfect them early on, and then use them as the next platform upon which to build even more complex motions. Biology calls these movements motor plans, and they possess a strong goal orientation. For instance, as infants we don't know how to walk, but we have a strong urge to keep moving in ways that strengthen and coordinate walking muscles and a strong desire to pull ourselves up and take steps. In humans, motor plans urge us to favor movements that will serve our best interests throughout our life. Some of our favorite motor plans develop from the basic motions of reaching, pulling, grasping, and pushing, for instance.

One of the best ways to get good at a complex action (such as playing a musical instrument or pitching a baseball game) is to practice it until it becomes a motor plan. Throwing the ball or playing musical scales over and over starts to feel almost automatic, able to be done quickly, almost effortlessly. With the motor plan in place, we can concentrate on the small but tricky adjustments that turn a fastball into a curveball or successive notes into a melody. This is where most of our movement habits come from, and as we know, habits have an upside and a downside. Motor plans are designed to be enduring, semiautomatic, and cost-effective. It's hard to break a bad habit because it's a motor plan. As the old saying goes, habits are the best servants and the worst masters.

Interestingly, the motor plan concept forms the basis for some theories of addiction. Some researchers have said that the bodily basis for addiction is a "programmed reach"; we see the doughnut and before we realize it, our arm has reached out to grasp it, pull it toward us, and put it in our mouth. This is the reasoning behind not having an open bag of potato chips at the couch, not putting yourself near drug paraphernalia, or putting a small portion of food on your plate and not taking seconds.

Motor plans make our lives a lot easier. Motor plans even get involved in procedures we set up, such as bedtime rituals where we always floss after brushing and before washing our hands. It may be that people in long-term relationships create motor plans among themselves—shared motor plans—though this idea hasn't been well researched. It would explain, however, the beauty of watching the members of a basketball team as they move in a coordinated dance toward the hoop. It's likely involved in why babies prefer their parents to hold them, as they have already developed shared motor plans that represent the physicality of attachment. It might also explain the ways couples who have been together a long time start to work together without the need for much talking.

Learning a new motor plan, whether we are nine months or ninety years old, involves attention, arousal, and emotion. In other words, if we start to practice a movement skill when we are tense and fearful, the tension and fear can become part of the plan. Our body's learning systems absorb all our present conditions when creating a motor plan, so if we practice with a tense body, we will tend to repeat the action with more tension than it needs. Because graceful and efficient motor plans have been so essential to our evolutionary survival, nature has paired them with play behavior in childhood. In this way we learn many of our motor plans during relatively safe, fun, and "pretend" circumstances. This reality should turn all of us into activists for early childhood playgrounds, keeping children away from TVs and cell phones until they are older, and including plenty of recess in school. This also speaks to the idea that bodyfulness can be a play practice as well as a contemplative one. From a bodyfulness perspective, it's never too late to have a playful childhood.

We need to develop as well as amend and dissolve motor plans throughout our lives. Developing them requires dedicated, conscious practice, as does amending and dissolving them. The good news is that bodyfulness practices can help with this because of their attention to the details of motor plans. Other contemplative practices, such as walking meditation, likely work in this way; the practitioner slows down their walk so that they can pay attention to the exquisite detail of taking each step. Staying awake and attentive during a motor plan allows it to be altered over time. Inhibiting an automatic motor plan very consciously—looking at the cigarette pack and feeling your arm not reaching for it, over and over—can also help lessen its grip on us. This same principle applies to people working with post-traumatic stress disorder (PTSD), where a trauma response, instead of resolving over time, becomes a motor plan and causes PTSD sufferers to repeat actions (such as cringing, startling, or panicking) that no longer apply to present circumstances. Increasingly, therapies for people with PTSD involve attending to the body, slowing down its movements while paying careful attention to them, and making new choices about how the movement sequences, as well as absorbing current, more emotionally positive circumstances into the motor plan.

Motor plans get started via lots of conscious attention and practice, and they continue by needing less and less. How we use our attention when we move, and how we attend to our movement, therefore becomes pivotal in the practice of bodyfulness.

Motor Plans Practice

One way to get started with this type of movement is to play with some of the fundamental actions that motor plans are built on, to see how they feel and what they bring up. Let's build on the reaching we did in a previous chapter. You can reach with various parts of your body, but the most common reach happens with the arms. Go ahead and reach, using one or both arms. Play for a minute with different kinds of reaches, ones that express different intentions or emotions, such as an insistent reach, an imploring reach, or a half-hearted reach. What images, memories, or feelings come up with each of these reaches? Take some time to acknowledge the associations that arise and past events that they might be holding. Now slow it way down. Reach out very slowly, noticing each individual muscle as it engages and disengages. Notice the weight of your arms and the path through space they take as they extend. Pay close attention to the process of reaching, and, if possible, play with reaching differently than you might usually. As much as possible, keep your attention on the details of the act of reaching, and experiment with altering those details consciously, just for fun. If it isn't fun or interesting, you may want to find someone to be with you and help you with this process. You don't have to do it alone or without the help of a professional, such as a body-centered psychotherapist.

You can continue this exercise with other fundamental movements, such as grasping, pulling, or letting go,[1] or with basic motor plans, such as walking or riding a bike. (Please keep yourself safe—don't play in traffic!) It might be useful to write down the different associations that come up with each movement, and then practice the movement again in fun, interesting, or companionable circumstances.

Another way to play with motor plans is to put on some music with a good beat to it and dance to the rhythms of the music. Let your body motions *agree* with the beats as much as possible, having fun with the synchronicity between you and the music. As an experiment, you can try to *clash* your motions with the music and pay attention to what happens. For extra credit, you can add in some of the motor plans we mentioned—pushing, reaching, pulling, walking, and so forth. Have fun!

Nonverbal Communication

Our next area of focus on the continuum of movement involves actions that become quite familiar and can be somewhat automatic. However, these actions have a lot more freedom than motor plans to be tweaked and played with and a lot more complexity. They have to do with the moving body's power to communicate.

Called nonverbal communication (NVC), this way of moving represents our first language, one we start to learn even in utero. When attuned caregivers respond to infants' expressive actions, the infants begin to learn that their smiles and cries mean something to others. They begin to use these movements purposefully, as do their caregivers, in order to make themselves understood and cared for with increasing levels of mutual complexity. From here, our first language—movement—is born.

We all consciously get the basics of NVC in pretty straightforward ways. We salute, we wrinkle our nose in disgust, and we smile broadly, fairly secure that these signals will be understood correctly. But NVC goes beyond these simplicities; it extends itself into emotions, culture, gender, social class, and power dynamics. Even though we learn the basics of a verbal language within a few years of birth, we continue to use our first, nonverbal language the rest of our lives, often layered onto our words as we speak them. When our verbal and nonverbal utterances are in lockstep, others often experience us as honest and trustworthy. But if we grit our teeth, squeeze our hands into fists, and growl out that we are *not* angry, then our listeners have a dilemma, and they usually believe what our body is doing rather than the words we are saying.

This is because verbal and nonverbal languages are specialized. Body language excels at communicating emotions, intentions, social status, sexuality, gender, communal affiliations, and power preferences. Verbal language tends to specialize in expressing our thinking, in talking about events in the past or the future, and in dealing with abstractions.

We first learn our body language at home, and as our world expands, we learn from friends, schools, social groups, and large systems (such as the army or social media). Because humans are a highly social species, we tend to succeed in life when we become good communicators in both verbal and nonverbal language systems. We move and belong to movement communities as much as we speak and belong to speech communities. Most of this first movement language, however, gets automatized and sinks below our conscious monitoring, running on its own.

Our emotional intelligence, however, is mostly measured by how in touch we are with our feeling, moving, and communicating body. When we want to know how we *really feel*, we typically need to check in with what we are *really doing*—our breathing pace and pattern, the tension in our face, the tone of our voice, the flutters in our stomach. The same goes for our ability to read others' body language. Without realizing it, we often notice a tiny movement in our friend's face or a tilt of their head, or hear that slight tremor in their voice, before we ask, "Are you really okay?" This sensitivity can be one of the definitions of a good friend.

Movement as Communication Practice

While it can be important to be able to disguise how we really feel—a need for safety or a desire for privacy, for example—in general, we do best when our verbal and nonverbal languages agree with each other and complement each other. (A lot of humor depends on a mismatch between verbal and nonverbal channels—very funny!)

This practice begins with knowing how you really feel, and knowing your feelings depends on reading your body. Begin with attending to the inner movements of your body, especially when you are in social settings. As much as possible over the next few days, consciously attend to your body while you are interacting with others and notice the small details of sensations. Think of these sensations as your body commenting on what is being said and not said in the room. Don't try to interpret your body by immediately creating a verbal translation of the sensation. Just notice the sensations, the emotions, and the patterns of tension in your body. Trust that this is a part of you that is speaking and that deserves your attention.

Another practice is to simply play more with communicating nonverbally. Whether it involves a good game of charades or playing with a friend, see if there are ways to express yourself just as well, or even better, nonverbally. Again, this often works best when we communicate feelings and emotions.

When you are listening to someone as they communicate with you, especially when they are sharing something personal, take some time to consciously attend to the small micromovements in their face, the subtle variations in their voice tone, and their posture and gestures. Don't try to interpret these messages yourself or assume you now know how they feel but use them to frame your questions and your communications to this person. Often just being sensitive to the fact that someone is feeling something can be enough for both of you to feel connected.

Spontaneous Movement

Our last big category of movement speaks to the more creative and spontaneous parts of ourselves. As we migrate toward the right-hand side of the movement continuum, our movement becomes less constrained, more adaptive to the details of present circumstances, and more unique. We see it in children as they cavort in the yard, in the abstracted motions of people dancing to rock and roll, or in any circumstance where we don't much plan what our body will do next. We might call it non-goal-oriented movement, physical motion done strictly for the sake of doing it. Often this is where movement-based art is born, as with a dancer in a studio trying out lots of different spontaneous actions until gradually favored ones are repeated, refined, and reproduced.

Spontaneous motion, of course, rests on the support of the previous actions—reflexes, motor plans, nonverbal communication. Only when these previous actions are relatively secure can we make use of our natural ability to be physically creative. How important is physical creativity? Likely, it's not going to kill us to refrain from creative movement. It may, however, limit our problem-solving skills, cause us to decline faster in old age, and inhibit our happiness. Challenging both the brain and the rest of the body with novelty, particularly physical novelty, has been shown to be one of our most effective antiaging regimens. Not only does this type of movement bring more blood (and therefore oxygen) to the brain (most forms of movement will do that, however), but it also contributes to neurogenesis, or the growth of new brain cells, which doesn't happen when movement is more habitual. This likely occurs because we have to pay attention while doing the action.

"Attention during action" may be one of our most succinct and poetic definitions of bodyfulness.

Experimenting outside the box of our habitual movement practices also tends to be fun, and having fun correlates to neurogenesis as well as to happiness. Physical play, even though it's non–goal oriented, has been shown to coordinate reflexes into motor plans, motor plans into NVC, and all of these into creative actions. Play also teaches us how to be in relationships and groups by helping us practice interacting, especially in the nonverbal realms of expressing and reading emotion.

Creativity researchers explore this idea of novelty, noting that not only art but also business, science, engineering, and other hard disciplines thrive through innovation. Problems become intractable when they can't be solved with well-known solutions, yet we keep trying those same old solutions. In these cases, stepping outside the box of habit, precedence, and received wisdom becomes essential. This departure from the way we usually see and do things is what made Albert Einstein famous, for instance. The concept of bodyfulness suggests that one of our best ways to cultivate out-of-the-box thinking is to practice out-of-the-box moving. Did you know that when Einstein was working on reinventing our relationship to time and space, he challenged himself by playing new and difficult music on his violin?

Creative Movement Practice

It can be tricky to step outside the box of the way we usually move. Let's start simply, with putting on some music, or if you are very brave, you can do this without music. Have some fun and just dance to the music, avoiding as much as possible any fixed moves. It may be advisable to do this alone, as you may get self-conscious about how you look when you dance, and dealing with self-consciousness may be too much extra effort at this point. The idea is to move how you feel rather than doing set moves. Often one of the best strategies at this point is to allow yourself to feel goofy; goofiness may be a sign that you are outside the box of the way you usually act.

Social dance movements have a lot more to do with being a member of a group than we realize. It's easy in the presence of others to automatically generate movements that send nonverbal signals to others. Dancing by ourselves, with no one there to "read" our body, can liberate spontaneous movement. The trick is to not feel bound to moving predictably or looking a particular way. It's just moving for the sake of enjoying the movement.

The next step in the practice is to use music that has no particular beat, so that you are not compelled to repeat the musical rhythms.

The next step after that is to lose the music completely and simply listen to your body as a way to generate your next actions. It works best when it's fun or enjoyable.

The next segment of this practice gets a bit more esoteric, but hang in there. You are going to work with your lower arm. To begin, just take a moment to move your hand and wrist around, loosening it up in any way that feels right. When you feel ready, go ahead and move your hand, wrist, and elbow very deliberately, very consciously, noticing the details of the experience. See if you can be attentive to the movement without having a sense of where it will go next, for maybe five minutes. For example, when you start curling your fingers in, you may predictably follow this movement through to making a fist. See if you can thwart this predictability: as soon as you notice that you can predict where the movement will go next, stop the movement and wait until another impulse arises, or just start doing a different action. You may be surprised at how frequently your will or your habits drive your actions.

This exercise plays with interrupting your will, gently and experimentally, and moving without a goal or plan. Don't worry if this proves difficult at first, just stay at it and play with it. The advanced practice involves doing this with your whole body.

We have now covered the basics of the mobility gradient, our continuum of movement. A word of caution: It can be seductive to imagine that creative movement is somehow a pinnacle of achievement, an end to which we aspire, yet this notion can unbalance us. Going back to our core principle of oscillation, we can see that bodyful movement covers the whole continuum, back and forth, in ways that celebrate the automatic as well as the spontaneous. Life requires all these movements. By moving purposefully along the continuum, in accordance with the meaningfulness we find in each of these actions, we can locate our bodyfulness in our present circumstances rather than striving for a seemingly ideal state that isn't meant to exist without its embodied companions on the continuum.

Stability and Mobility in Movement

If we take a step back and look at the whole mobility gradient, a few overarching principles emerge, such as stability and mobility. Stability keeps us grounded, rooted, and supported. Mobility enables us to change our location and go after things. We need both.

Looking metaphorically at the two, how would you characterize your current status with stability and mobility? How do these two principles live in your body? In your psyche? Often in a complex action we hold one part of our body stable while another moves, like a dancer standing on one leg while raising and gesturing with the other. Injuries tend to occur when one part of the body becomes overmobile or overstabile compared to its neighbors, creating a conflict. Bodyfulness allows the stable parts of ourselves to work in tandem with the mobile areas. Again, both work best when supported by the other. Mobility and stability don't have to be fifty-fifty; sometimes our lives impel us to settle down more, and other times life urges us to wander. The bodyfulness practice is to find stability within mobility, and mobility within stability.

Stability and Mobility Practice

Starting with stability, let's experiment with a sitting meditation posture, if you are able. Sit on something such as a cushion or the front portion of a chair seat without back support, and sense your spine as both upright and relaxed. Spend some time in this relative stillness, noticing your body. Which areas seem to grip more to hold yourself up, and which don't seem to be working at all? Even when no discernible movement occurs, micromovements happen both inside various parts of your body as well as your whole body, which sways ever so slightly. Notice these small movements, such as your breathing and heartbeat, as well as the contraction of muscles in your torso and neck. Take some moments to play with how these small motions might support your body's stability. Did any associations come up? Note these. Stability becomes stronger, with less effort, when we slightly contract the small muscles around our spine to keep us stable, instead of recruiting the big muscles close to the surface of our body. The big muscles only come into play as stabilizers if we do something really mobile, such as throw a ball. Take some time to imagine these small, short muscles as they span one vertebra to the next. It can take some practice to get more in touch with them, but once you do, you may feel as though your spine can lengthen by floating up a few centimeters rather than having to be pushed up in a tense way by larger muscles.

For our mobility practice, two types of motion can help: wiggling and stretching. Wiggling loosens our joints and stretching loosens our muscles. Both help us be mobile. As much as you are able, play with wiggling and stretching in various positions: sitting, standing, bending over, lying down. Just do as much as feels right, making up stretches and wiggles that feel good to you. Notice the parts of your body that stabilize so that the other parts can move. What associations come up when you play with getting more mobile? Does anything about these associations feel applicable to your daily life?

Kinesphere

Our next bodyfulness movement principle takes up the issue of space—the space we move in and through, called our kinesphere. Imagine it as a bubble around each of us that marks the limits of how far we can extend, reach, or gesture in the space. We tend to lay claim to this space as ours and only let into it the people whom we feel safe with or close to. Sometimes we use all of it, such as when we yawn and stretch, and sometimes just parts of it, such as when reading a book. Again, metaphors arise. How much space is it okay for you to take up in the world? What associations do you have to "taking up a lot of space" or using just a portion of the space around you?

Cultures tend to codify how their members use space as an experience and expression of identity and community. For example, how space is used can signal gender roles in many cultures. How we move exists in a network of mutual influences between how much effort we use, how much speed we use, and how much space we take up, and these are all molded by the systems we live in, such as families, communities, and societies. People who move differently than the privileged norms (such as white, straight, able-bodied, middle-class movement) can be punished or ostracized. Bodyfulness can help us examine our use of space and consciously test how we want to live in as well as challenge our society.

Kinesphere Practice

Playing with your kinesphere can be pretty straightforward. Start with an image of a bubble around you. Play with reaching out to touch the borders of it with various body parts, and then see how small you can get inside it. You can use music as a support, or not. What are the images, sounds, emotions, and memories that come up when you reach out and pull into the space? Do any old rules come up, such as "I'm not supposed to get big" or "I'm not supposed to get small"? Notice the norms you may have absorbed about how you use the space around you. You don't necessarily have to change them, but it can be an important self-reflection to know they are there and to make conscious choices about them.

Power

Lastly, and perhaps most importantly, our status on the mobility gradient illuminates one of our most fundamental life issues: power. Movement literally em*power*s us; it expresses our power or ability to do what we can do. Whether we are moving in a wheelchair or on our feet, our ability to get from here to there signifies our successful efforts to act on what we feel or want. This completes the sensorimotor loop we spoke of before: I feel, and I act on what I feel. Interestingly, evolution has set us up so that when we organize and complete movement sequences that are related to our feelings or wants, our brain secretes a bit of dopamine (a neurotransmitter associated with pleasure) that helps us feel satisfied and positive about what we just did. This explains our pleasure at quenching our thirst, which involves reaching for the glass of water, grasping it, pulling it toward us, and swallowing the water within it. This small, everyday act contributes to our more global sense of empowerment: how I move gets me what I want or need in small but cumulative ways, over and over.

Psychologists have specialized phrases for these experiences of empowerment—*self-efficacy*, *a sense of agency*, and *internal locus of control*, for example—and see the lack of these as contributing to depression, helplessness, anxiety, and aggression. These terms are not related to a feeling that "I'm in charge or in control of everything" but rather that I basically steer my course in life. This also relates to the central prayer of 12-step programs that asks our higher power for the courage to change the things we can, to accept the things we can't change, and to have the wisdom to know the difference. Psychotherapy, in fundamental ways, seeks to help people find a right relationship to self-empowerment.

As a term applied to individuals as well as families, cultures, systems, and societies, *power* can be neutral (the power of a lever to lift something), positive (the power to do good), or negative (the abuse of power). Our models for how to use our power begin in our earliest relationships and continue throughout our lifetime, changing like the tide with age, events, and relationships. Good parenting involves helping our children experience the shifting range of their power, such that they learn to manage all the ways that power occurs. This facilitates learning skills related to times when we are not in control; it's vital to our well-being that we make peace with situations where our actions will not bring about desired results or when what we want turns out not to be a good idea. This parallels the mobility gradient itself, where some movements lie outside our will and control, some are partially within our control, and others are completely within our control.

Our relationship to power all boils down to moving, or kinetic energy. My movements generate sensations, these sensations tell me how I feel, and from there I can reflect on and know what I want. It remains for me to move as a means of enabling these things. When I can "make it happen" fairly consistently (but not constantly), I feel more able to make choices about who I am and what happens to me.

Our relationship to power is yet another continuum: at one extreme we feel powerless, and at the other extreme we feel all-powerful. While life can sometimes thrust us into either extreme, our contentment likely lies in an oscillation that enjoys and occupies the middle range. Purposeful moving can help us find our way on this oscillation.

Powerfulness Practice

The word *power* carries rich associations, and these associations can tell us a lot about our history with how power has played out in our lives. Take a few minutes to write down a few associations that occur to you when you say the word *power*. Just note down whatever words, images, sounds, memories, or feelings come up when you contemplate that word. Then look at your list. What kinds of themes seem to be there in the list?

Now use your body to work with those words. Pick a word from your list and say it either to yourself or out loud. Hold the word in your careful attention for a bit, then notice how your body responds to the word. Does it start to slump, to tingle, to rise up? Is there no particular reaction? Whatever response you notice, just allow it to happen, perhaps supporting it to become more visible. You may experience a body memory—when your body physically enacts its memories of how power works, for you and the people around you. These body memories can make the past seem very real and present because your body is doing them now. Does it feel right to keep doing these body memories? In what ways do these sensations and movements support or inhibit your current well-being?

Ideally we want to use our power wisely, neither abdicating nor abusing it, and behaving in ways that allow us to accomplish our work, such as cooking dinner, going to school, or asking for assistance with our care and mobility.

In many cases we need support and help with empowerment, whether that involves working with a therapist, a community organization, a political party, or a friend. Many of us have been traumatized by abuses of power. Many of us haven't examined the ways in which we have abused our power or taken for granted the power that a privileged status has afforded us. For these reasons, you may not want to do these practices by yourself, and opt instead for the support and challenge of having people around you. Power exists in relationship to people and things and can ultimately only be worked with in relationship to them.

Exercise and Body Tone

Related to the idea of power, bodyfulness can be enhanced by developing more conscious control of our moving body. We frequently use the word *tone* for this, as we saw in the section on hypertone, tone, and hypotone. Tone happens when we perform an action in the Goldilocks zone—the action uses just the right amount of strength, not too much and not too little. Exercise increases our resting body tone, particularly in our postural muscles, and our sense of feeling fit. Just leading an active lifestyle, whatever that means for your particular body, increases your tone. Good posture and the ability to pay attention often are results of good body tone. Research has validated the strong relationship between good postural tone and attentional clarity and focus, and the ability to focus our attention is strongly correlated to intelligence, creativity, and healthy aging. This likely explains why most meditation traditions work with creating a good meditation posture as a vital part of the practice.

Whatever our state of physical ability, whatever fitness looks like in our body, tone is a state that pervades all our interdependent systems—physical, mental, and emotional. While this isn't a new idea, how we apply it to bodyfulness *is* new. Fitness used to be thought of as exercise and diet, such as calisthenics and eating your vegetables. When we include a more full-bodied and contemplative perspective, we can see fitness as moving the body in ways that challenge it, and the challenge involves novelty, creativity, and moment-to-moment engagement with all the senses. Pedaling on an exercise bike while checking our emails likely generates some benefit, but it's not cultivating bodyfulness.

Bodyfulness in relation to tone means being awake as we move. It means attending as fully as possible to what we are doing—our breathing, our sensing, and our relationship to our environment—in an atmosphere of physical challenge. How might that show up for you? Going out dancing? A yoga class? A brisk walk on a cold morning? Learning a new sport? It could be through any number of different activities. The physical challenge should be tailored to your body and your circumstances and can involve almost anything, as long as it doesn't get rote or too predictable. Its core features should involve something that you have to pay attention to in order to keep doing it and something that, while challenging your breathing and your strength, should be basically pleasant to do. If you combine the intentions of contemplative practice with actions that often make you sweat, you are there.

Fitness Practice

It may be interesting to play a bit more with the neutral and pragmatic manifestations of power—defined as the ability to do work or the rate at which work is done. Our question revolves around whether or not we can produce sufficient strength or endurance to accomplish tasks we care about, such as increasing health or well-being, preventing age-related decline, or maintaining the strength to pick up and hold a child.

Choose the exercise yourself, so that you can experiment with actions that make you physically stronger over time. First make sure that you and/or your doctor feel that you are up for it. Then pick a regimen that targets some kind of strength building and balances muscle groups such as flexors and extensors (such as toning your back and abdomen or your hip flexors and your hip extensors). Make sure the exercise and regimen are simple, sustainable, and adaptable. This is strength training, and you are playing with the notion that physical strength often relates to psychological strength. Pay attention to the act of doing it as a contemplative practice. When you exercise this way, note how you feel during and afterward as well as over the longer haul. It's very common that with consistent strength training we feel "better," whether that be a better mood, more energy, or better sleep. But also notice if you feel more capable, more able to manage things, more emotionally strong. While this correlation may not be true for everyone, it might be worth the time and energy to experiment with it, since playing with our body's tone via physical strength disciplines carries so much inherent benefit for most of us.

Another way to work with body tone is to gain more control of your ability to let go of it, technically called hypotone. We all know that feeling when we feel tense somewhere and can't let it go. This is called structural holding, or hypertone, an ongoing tension that we are not able to release. Functional holding, on the other hand, occurs when we feel a contracted muscle and just let it go when we don't need to use it anymore.[2] We want to be able to restore functional holding so that structural holding doesn't keep us chronically tense. Again, tone lies on a continuum, from the extreme of hypotone, which involves not being able to accomplish something in motion, into the large middle ground of tone, and to the other extreme of hypertone, where our excessive tension can get in the way of completing an action. Conscious practice along this continuum can help us lead a bodyful and "toned" life.

One of the best strategies to use here comes from the practice of progressive relaxation, developed by Edmund Jacobson. He was one of the first physicians to notice that as we let go of muscular contraction our attention wanes (like when we fall asleep) and that contracting muscles tends to sharpen attention. He also pioneered the ideas that the nervous system wakes up, sharpens attention, and increases body tone when novelty occurs and that we only have control over muscles that we can feel. His progressive relaxation practice leverages these concepts by noting that in order to gain control over the ability to let go of a muscle, we need to first wake up the nervous system by creating a contrast, in this case by *increasing* a muscle contraction first, which gives us more proprioceptive feeling and therefore more ability to let go of the tension.

Relaxation Practice

This exercise is best done lying comfortably on a carpeted floor or a mat. It's also best if you start at your feet and work systematically up your body, all the way from feet to head, but you decide where is best to start. You can also do a short form by identifying a tense muscle and just working there.

Begin by noticing any tension you feel in various parts of your body. Just notice. Then put your attention to your ankles. Flex your ankles, so that your toes come closer to your head. Take a moment to really feel exactly where you are contracting in order to accomplish this action. Which muscles are in use? Hold the tension, feeling it for a bit, then let it go, let it relax. Feel the weight of your feet, and as much as possible let their weight sink into the floor for a bit. Repeat the contraction a few times, each time identifying the working muscle, releasing the tension, and feeling the weight after the release. Repeat this process in all your major joints. Often you need only to lift a body part off the floor, just slightly, to contract a muscle. Letting go just allows it to fall back to the floor. See if you can keep letting go, even more, as you practice. Don't be surprised if you get sleepy. This can be a good thing. If you doze off, no worries.

Conscious movement practices come in a variety of forms, as they pick up many of the important themes and metaphors that moving brings us. The word *movement* holds many meanings: getting from here to there, feeling emotional in response to experiencing something, changing something, or organizing activism. When we move, we bring up and enact various memories of how life has moved us and how we have moved through it. All these relationships to movement deserve to be engaged with and made as conscious as possible in a bodyful life. Movement also brings us closer to and farther away from others, and it's this application to relationships that we will play with in the next chapter.

6

Relating

HUMANS ARE SOCIAL. As a species we are drawn to live in groups, to feel happier when we are connected to others, and to feel lonely when we go too long without relational contact. We group together for purposes of mutual safety, comfort, caring, stimulation, and cooperation. Because of the core nature of these purposes, most of our imprints about relationships are laid down very early, in the crucible of our nonverbal, body-to-body, and emotional interactions—how we were held, gazed at, spoken to as a young child.

These early bodily experiences with our caregivers matter because they imprint automatic habits in our body that impel our adult thoughts and behaviors. These body habits endure as physical tendencies in subsequent relationships, as proclivities to move in certain ways when we are in contact with others. We may not even realize that we have a habit of shrinking in the presence of people with more status or power, or that we gravitate toward people who vaguely resemble our mother, or that we hold our breath when we feel attracted to someone. These physical movements give us the impression that the current interaction is similar to old ones.

No matter what our childhood was like, our task as adults is to keep practicing and refining healthy relational skills and to actively push back against our own relational tendencies that hurt us and others or cause us to lose connection. Bodyfulness involves working with our difficult enduring tendencies through moving, breathing, and sensing differently within our current relationships. Bodyfulness literally touches into the blood and guts of what it means to be a relational creature. This may be why it may not suffice to sit on a meditation cushion, mindfully, in order to get better at relationships. The core of our being isn't just ours alone but binds itself together with others, ancestrally and currently. In a very real way we become who we are *interactionally*, through what we do together with others and how we feel in the doing.

The Semipermeable Relationship

We saw in chapter 2 that our body's cells operate with semipermeable boundaries that on a moment-to-moment basis allow some things in and out, and not others. This mechanism of balancing discernment with access to resources, as well as identity with exchange, ensures our well-being by creating important interdependencies among our cells. Our body ends up a cooperative jumble of trillions of internal relationships.

As inside, so outside. Our body relates to countless external elements—air, water, trees, animals, the built environment, other humans—and we can't exist without them. This is what Buddhist monk Thich Nhat Hanh means when he talks about interbeing, as we covered in chapter 2. Sooner or later we relate to and exchange with all existence, so much so that it's hard not to think of us as also a cooperative jumble of trillions of external relationships. Yet here we are, having ongoing experiences of being a separate self.

While it can be fun and deeply meaningful to contemplate the nature of existence, let's look for a bit at the more mundane issues in our relationships, the ones we have at home, at work, and at the grocery store. Extending our cellular metaphor, a relationship only becomes possible when a boundary forms that creates an entity that can then "relate to" other entities. Boundaries hold things together; they hold *me* together. We typically think of boundaries as keeping things separate, but we can now see this idea is a bit shortsighted. A boundary *regulates* identity. And our boundaries regulate our relationships.

When we say yes or no to something, we are regulating our boundaries, either softening them or firming them up. When we get close enough to touch someone, or distant enough to lose track of them, we are altering our boundaries. Bodyfulness takes advantage of this ongoing natural process and leverages it, asking us to become more aware of our discernment and to engage with it more consciously through the body.

Again, the body's middle path guides us. A border that dissolves too readily or firms up too strongly will soon inhibit both discernment and exchange. Life seems to require that we oscillate along a continuum, where rare moments of *fusion* and *isolation* bracket an extensive middle ground of *contact*. To be in contact with someone (or something) means we are in touch with them, we are exchanging with them. This seems to be the place where relationships work their magic.

When a boundary isn't strong enough for current circumstances —during a perceived threat, for instance—we shore it up and become defensive. Defending ourselves can quite literally save our lives in extreme cases. Yet often we become defensive when we don't need to, when it actually gets in the way of healthy contact. When a boundary is too strong for current circumstances—during a loving touch, for instance—we can learn to loosen it and become open and vulnerable. Becoming more open can also save our lives, in a way. Yet often we can become vulnerable in ways and at times that are harmful to ourselves or others and get in the way of being contactful. Our practice involves increasing our flexibility and discernment around being in contact in our relationships.

Conscious Borders Practice

Take a few contemplative moments to sit quietly and notice your body's borders. You can feel them acutely when they are in contact with a surface, such as the couch or your clothing. You might even be able to feel them through your skin's contact with the air. Take another few moments to oscillate your attention from inside you to outside you, and then attend to the surface of your body. Stay with this oscillation for some minutes, and then, if possible, spend some time noticing what associations come up—sensations, images, feelings, memories—as you pay attention to your borders. Greet these associations and, without analysis or judgment, hold them in your attention. Later you might want to reflect on the associations, seeing them as possible traces from earlier interactions.

Relational Touch

Physical touch ranks as one of our finest means of experiencing contact. In childhood, touch is so necessary that young children can experience lasting brain damage or even die from its absence.[1] Metaphoric touch—when we speak of being touched by someone emotionally or talk about our gazes touching—expands our repertoire of contactfulness. This fundamental need for physical and metaphoric contact creates complex terrains because touch not only communicates affection, love, support, healthy sexuality, and nurturance, but also disapproval, control, violence, and dominance. Most of us have been touched in all these various ways. On top of this massive complexity, cultures and subcultures further complicate our understanding of touch. If we imagine all human cultures on a touch continuum, we can see there are "high touch" cultures all the way down to "low touch" cultures. Cultures also form elaborate rules about who can touch whom, where on the body, and under what circumstances. Just the gender politics of touch can be incredibly daunting.

Given that touch occurs at our borders and against our skin, and that we have to come into close proximity with someone's body in order to touch them, its position as a powerful relational force becomes clear. How can we heal our old touch wounds? What would it look like if we were to be more aware and respectful of people's touch history, their touch culture, and their touch boundaries? How can we touch ourselves and others in bodyful ways? Working on the answers to these questions augments our relational skills. It begins with self-touch and graduates to touch with others.

Touch Practice

Begin by finding a position that feels comfortable and contemplative, and then take a few minutes to feel your borders. Notice all the touching already going on—the passive touch of your clothing on your skin, parts of your body in contact with the floor or chair, the feel of the air on your skin—and notice any associations that arise. Greet them and keep them as part of what you are attending to. Now use your hands to actively touch some part of your body, such as your face or lower arms, where the contact can be skin to skin. Just notice the sensations the touch engenders. Experiment with different types of touch—a light stroking or a firm grip. Pay attention to any associations that arise. Greet these associations, and without analysis or judgment, hold them in your attention. Later you might want to reflect on the associations, seeing them as possible traces from earlier interactions.

In the next days and weeks, be more aware of your passive and active touching of others. Set an intention to be more conscious and purposeful about your touching (or not touching) and being touched. Notice the etiquette you use regarding touch and question it more: Do I initiate touch without really knowing if the person I'm touching wants it? Talk to friends and family about this topic, perhaps sharing stories of your touch histories or your observations about your historical or current touch cultures and how these cultures intersect when you touch each other. If possible, take time with a friend, a pet, or a loved one to touch very consciously, as a contemplative practice.

Bodily Attunement

In chapter 5, we looked at moving as a form of communication. Now we can add in a deeper appreciation of how movement manages moments of contact within relationships. From the vantage point of bodyfulness, much of our face-to-face relational communication is nonverbal. Understanding others and being understood by them across our semipermeable borders involves an ongoing and hopefully graceful body dance that remains unconscious most of the time. It's our job now to wake up to it more and consciously align it with our relational aspirations.

Communication can occur at two levels of sophistication: expression and attunement. When we express (*ex-press*, or "press out") ourselves, we send out a signal. Expression often remains a simple form of communication because it starts as something inside us that we are releasing out toward others, such as when we shout or a baby cries. Often this simplicity is quite sufficient, especially when we don't need a feeling of closeness with our listener. When we are just expressing what is inside of us, we may not particularly consider the person on the receiving end of the communication. A lot of relational discord can occur when we express ourselves and then become upset when we fail to feel understood, because in order to be deeply understood we usually need to shape our expressions to our listener, in a kind of *pas de deux* of reciprocal communication.

When we communicate in an attuned way, we consider who we are with. Are they young or old? Tired or anxious? Culturally different than us? Sexually attractive to us? We then shape our expressions (both the content and the delivery) into forms that are more likely to be understood by them. When we do this and our listener responds in a similar manner, we become attuned to each other, that delicious feeling of mutual sympathy, connectedness, and shared experiences. Shaping our expressions can certainly go too far, to the point where we mimic and therefore disrespect other people's expressive cultures or lose our sense of our own expressive culture. Again, attunement resides in a middle ground and in semipermeability. While attunement can't be and should not be constant (except, it seems, in romance novels), its presence does make life meaningful and loving.

As you would by now imagine, attunement occurs principally

through the body and originally through early nonverbal interactions with caregivers. It has to do with how much tension is in our body, how we shape our body as we communicate, where we set our gaze, and how close or far away we are. It also involves our posture, gestures, touch, speed and movement rhythms, and the quality of our voice tone. This can all be said to form our *body narratives*. We feel attuned to people who read and understand our body narratives and whose body narratives we take the time and effort to understand. On a conscious level, we like to be around these people, and we feel close to them.

Bodyfulness makes a contemplative practice out of attunement. How can I wake up to my body narratives and make them more understandable? How can I consciously get better at reading the body narratives of people with whom I feel close, so that I might feel attuned with them? When attunement is broken in normal relational conflicts, how can I work to get it back? We have been building up the answers to these questions, as they substantially involve being able to read our own subtle body states, from our inside sensations to our visible movements. When we are in tune with ourselves, we become more capable of tuning in to others. It only remains to practice and get better at sensing others' subtler body stories in the crucible of our current relationships.

Attunement Practices

- If you can, find a friend or loved one who is willing to experiment with you. Sit facing each other. Now, both of you oscillate between eyes open and looking at your partner and eyes closed and noticing what is going on in your body. When you attend inside, really notice the small happenings there. When your attention goes out to your partner, do the same, noticing small tensions, subtle leanings, or the details of their breathing. There will be times when your eyes are open and on each other at the same time and times when one or both of you will have eyes closed, or one of you will be looking while the other isn't. Just notice what associations come up under these different conditions:

- Eyes open and on the other, and their eyes are closed

- Eyes open and on the other, and their eyes are on you

- Eyes closed and you don't know if their eyes are on you or not

Each of these conditions can bring up relational issues. Is it okay to be visible to another? Is it okay to look at someone? Is it okay to not know if I'm being seen? Is it okay to not see someone else and spend time with myself? Is it okay if another person spends time with themselves and not with me? If you would like, when you end the exercise, talk it over with your partner: What were your associations to these different conditions? Particularly, what happened in your body in response to the different conditions? The observations will give you some clues as to your early and nonverbal imprints about relationships. The exercise will also give you some practice in sensing body states while in relationship.

- Either in a freestanding practice or embedded within ongoing interactions, take some moments in your day to pay greater attention to others' postures and gestures, and in particular to the looks on their faces. We read each other's bodies constantly but remain mostly unaware that we do so. We also tend to use these unconscious readings as a means of assessing their state, their intentions toward us, and their efforts at communication. By doing this consciously, and as a practice, we can surface old assumptions that might be more about us than about them. We can also get better at these readings, often by asking the person we are interacting with about how they are feeling. While there are times when we don't know how we really feel, or are used to misrepresenting how we feel, it can be important to be more conscious about these two streams of information: what is said and what is being expressed through the body.

- This exercise involves two people. It may be interesting to do it multiple times, once with a colleague, once with a friend, once with a family member. Stand facing each other and choose who will stand still while the other one moves. During the exercise, both partners will track their ongoing state, noticing sensations and other associations. Begin the first few minutes of the exercise without talking, but after some time either of you can share what you are noticing in yourself (just describe; don't interpret). Now, the mover can begin to experiment with getting closer to and farther away from their partner. What associations come up for you both at the different distances? Perhaps as your partner gets farther away, you feel a sense of relief or maybe a sense of being left behind. Try not to judge; just notice how getting closer and farther away affects you. The mover can play with approaching and retreating from different angles or at different speeds or levels. Just play with it. When you are ready to conclude the practice, take a few minutes to talk about it together. Then switch roles so that the mover becomes the stander. Notice if the associations change when your role changes. When you are ready to conclude the practice, talk again.

You can extend the exercise to allow both of you to move at the same time. Notice what happens in you when you both get closer at the same time or both get more separation. Notice what happens in you when one of you wants to get closer when the other wants to get farther away. When you finish, take a few minutes to discuss how the conditions in the exercise might have illustrated patterns you have in relationships.

The Coregulation of Relating Bodies

When we can consistently attune with someone we care about, we create a sphere of mutual influence between us. We affect each other, both in short-term moods and in long-term tendencies. One of the hallmarks of a good relationship might be that over time this influence tends to bring out the best in both partners: we listen to our spouse at the end of their stressful day, in a way that helps them relax; our calm assurances and enveloping embrace soothes a crying child; we encourage a sad friend to take a walk with us. This influence can also involve avoiding negatives—for example, we minimize excessive complaining so that we don't pull others down with us. And as we saw previously, this influence also consists of lessening attunement (firming up boundaries) when appropriate.

This influence is often called coregulation, and as you might imagine, it begins before birth and rests largely on the coregulation of physical states.[2] My calm body—my slow heart rate, my deep breathing, my relaxed tone—all help you feel better when I hug you at the end of a hard day. As a result, your heart rate likely lowers, your breath deepens, and your muscles relax. This coregulation happens within our body (our metabolism) and also between our bodies. Video research, for instance, has consistently shown that people who like each other tend to gesture synchronistically when they sit and talk together, a kind of nonverbal dance going on under the radar.[3]

Relational bodyfulness helps us wake up to this influence, get better at being a positive influence, and be more open to positive influences from others with whom we are in reciprocal relationships. As we have seen so many times before, this begins with our own ability to self-regulate. Can we calm ourselves down when distressed, without habitually needing drugs, alcohol, or the Internet? Can we cheer ourselves up? Can we experience sadness or anger as positive influences during trying times? Can we balance our breathing so that our whole metabolism becomes more regulated? Our primary job as adults is to empower ourselves in our own regulation so that we can bring ourselves back from dysregulated states and generate our own regulated states, using our body as the means. Only then can we become a positive influence for others.

One of the skills of coregulation is to learn the difference between influence and manipulation. We are certainly not the arbiters of what works for other people. It's not about trying to get them into another state that we deem better for them (or us) or requiring others to be our regulator. Nor is it about the self-manipulation of willing ourselves to do the right thing out of a critical vigilance. At its heart, bodyfulness is about attunement and enhancing our capacity to emotionally "know" others (and ourselves). When we act responsively to what or whom we are attuned to, coregulation can occur as a natural by-product—my feeling sad when my friend shares her grief, or excited at her triumphs, for instance. In other words, bringing bodyfulness to our relationships means practicing coregulation consciously. This practice shies away from specific or prescribed outcomes and works instead to experience shared states that help us feel closer, in ways that on the whole regulate all involved.[4]

Coregulation Practices

- Take some opportunities over the next few days to work consciously with your breathing, moving, and sensing body in situations where you would like to get better at self-regulation. While there are many extant practices that can help you with this, such as the balanced breathing practice or taking a walk after dinner, only you know what works. Trust yourself to adopt tried-and-true practices, adapt others, and make up others on your own. If possible, practice this body-based self-regulation during challenging situations. Make sure to practice both cultivating more positive states as well as bringing yourself back from stressful ones.

- Take some opportunities over the next few days to work consciously with others as a positive influence, body to body. This might involve being more present during a hug or taking a few deep, audible breaths when things get tense in a meeting, not as a way to get others to breathe more deeply or to reduce what may be needed tension in the group but as a way to help the tension be regulated enough to be productive.

Relational Play

One other childhood activity rivals early caregiver interactions as the builder of our relational world: play. So important is play that all mammals and birds engage in it, most for their whole lives. Play increases physical fitness, organizes the brain, relieves stress, teaches multiple skills, and cements learning. By its nature, play tends to be fun; it exists outside of a goal-directed day, allowing us to experiment with doing and saying things we might not normally risk.

For our purposes here, we want to investigate play's role in relationships. During childhood, play helps us learn the complex job of how be in relationships and how to be part of a group. In play we rehearse, experiment, and test the boundaries of nuanced social interactions.

Play helps us generate and share positive states with others, whether it be on a ball field, across a game board, or in a backyard. This link between feeling good and feeling connected to others likely has roots in our evolutionary past, where those who bonded and cooperated thrived. As you can now assume, relational play occurs in and through the body. Our first experiments in play are physical, and play remains largely physical throughout childhood, gradually expanding to include more cognitive forms such as humor and games with complex cognitive strategies. As adults, we also add in that very pinnacle of play—sex.

What if play could be contemplative? What would it look like if we engaged in physical and relational play as a bodyfulness practice? Certainly sex has been explored as a contemplative practice, especially in the East. If we define play as any activity done for no other purpose than the enjoyment of doing it, we have a broad canvas upon which to paint our bodyful states. Relational play, through the body, can help us wake up to and get better at contact, softening and firming our boundaries, attunement, and coregulation, all within the frame of positive experiences. It can be practiced as a freestanding activity and as an embedded attitude within our ongoing interactions. What makes play a bodyful practice is doing it while consciously breathing, moving, sensing, and relating, as well as supporting ourselves to fully participate in positive states, particularly those we can share with others.

Relational Play Practices

The following is a list of relational play practices you can use as a starting point. Ultimately you will design your own bodyful play. The goal of the practice is to play, be in contact with your playmates, and be bodyful at the same time. No small feat!

- Sit facing your playmate, and make gestures, faces, and sounds back and forth as a nonverbal, relational exchange.

- As a kind of charades, try to communicate something to a playmate using only sounds, gestures, looks, and postures.

- Move around (dancing or just spontaneously moving) while your playmate tries to accurately mirror the movement. Switch roles.

- Nonverbally try to get your playmate to laugh, without touching them. Switch roles.

- Recruit a child to run around with, taking their lead in the play experience.

Cocreated Bodyful States

Virtually all religious traditions value practicing together in community. Most of us have directly experienced the power of being together with others: moving, singing, meditating, or praying as a group. At times like these there seems to be an acceleration of feeling, a multiplier effect, helping us all practice more deeply. Whether we are practicing with one other person or thousands of others, in being together we can cocreate contemplative states. Cocreating bodyful states follows from this ancient human experience.

Just like it takes two to tango, cocreating bodyfulness requires attention to bodily relating. Yes, we still monitor and value our inner experience, but in this relational dance we create a kind of community body, one that operates as a co-op. Much like the tango, we practice moving together, anticipating, signaling, supporting, making up moves, and enjoying the results. We don't lose ourselves but rather temporarily expand our sense of who we are in order to include another. When this is done consciously and reflected upon, it becomes a bodyfulness practice.

Relational and Community Practice

- This exercise involves sitting meditation with one other person, and it involves touch. To begin, sit shoulder to shoulder. Take a few minutes first to sit quietly on your own, practicing a form of sitting meditation familiar to you.[5] Then one of you reaches your arm behind your partner and rests your hand on the middle or the small of their back. The other partner does the same. Over the next several minutes (you decide how long), both of you oscillate your attention between your bodily experience and what you can feel of your partner's body from your touch and proximity. You might be able to feel their breathing or small movement adjustments. Just be with these small states, both with yourself and with your partner. You may notice moments of synchrony, such as breathing together, or you may notice a lot of difference between the two of you. It isn't about being the same but rather being together. Either way, just notice and be with your body without judgment or explanation.

- This exercise can also be done sitting side by side, perhaps six inches separating your shoulders. When ready, lean toward one another, and take a few moments to lean into each other, sharing your weight together. Notice how this feels. Then one of you just gives your weight to the other, for the other to hold (this may require more than shoulders, but you both can decide how this happens). Both of you notice how this feels, what associations come up with it. Switch roles, with the other partner giving all their weight for the other to hold. Talk about it afterward. Did any images come up related to sharing, giving, and holding another's weight?

- Just a recommendation, if you are in a position to do so: Think about taking a partner-based dance class. Nothing surfaces relationship issues better than having to move together with someone in a coordinated fashion. Bonus feature: research on aging notes that couples dancing can ward off cognitive decline due to the triple whammy of sharpening attention, promoting physical well-being, and fostering social connection.

The four core practices in this section of the book—breathing, moving, sensing, and relating—work together to help us stay awake to our direct, lived experiences. By working synergistically, they support us in our wakefulness to stay engaged with all manner of life events, from painful to pleasurable, mundane to life changing. The result of this bodyful connectedness means that both the information and the resources inherent in these powerful life functions can be available to us in each moment.

PART THREE

Bodyful Applications and Actions

Body Identity, Body Authority, and Bodyful Stories

"Who am I?" constitutes one of our most fundamental human questions and can engender a tremendous amount of late-night angst as well as contemplative curiosity. In the introduction to this book I offered a rather simplistic answer: we are a body. Let's "flesh out" a more nuanced answer at this point and see how our bodily sense of self is related to bodyfulness. Once again, this exploration will involve oscillation and attention as well as breathing, moving, sensing, and relating.

We often wrestle with "Who am I?" as a question of identity. Early psychological theory tended to assume that identity development provided one with a singular sense of unity and purpose, that it formed in childhood, was complete by adulthood, and stayed much the same after that. In this scenario, who we are tends to be measured first physically (gender, weight, reflexes, behavioral abilities), but as we mature, cognitive development becomes more and more important, so much so that it's seen as separate from the body. As a result, the sense of self we finally arrive at is largely mental; we become our mind and what we think, more or less. That is who we are, at least from a classical standpoint.

Current developmental theorists tend to challenge this trajectory. They note that our concept of identity needs to accommodate multiplicity, conflict, and even contradiction in the structure of the self. They assert that we don't need to assume a singular identity or even a fixed sense of self. This view dovetails with many contemplative traditions that question the existence of a solid self. The theorist Hubert ("Bert") J. M. Hermans, for instance, talks about our taking different "I" positions. He states that "the I fluctuates along different and even opposed positions, and can give each position a voice so that they can talk/relate to each other. Each voice has a story to tell about his or her own experiences, from his or her own stance, resulting in a complex narratively structured self."[1] Several other theorists call this our narrative identity and see it as comprising the stories we tell about ourselves and the stories that others tell about us. Once these stories become solidified by being retold, we tend to believe them, and then we tend to live by them.

These changing and multiple selves, constructed via our repeated and reinforced stories, possess both toxic and redemptive possibilities. We all understand the effects that can result when as children we are shamed or denigrated and how this can manifest in our adult view of ourselves. We can also see the same toxic effects on a systemic level, where people of color, for instance, are repeatedly exposed to media and people who tell them they are worthless, that they are problematic. Our health and illnesses may also be linked to these stories. Psychotherapy often involves reconfiguring our stories as a way to work through old, internalized negative narratives and find redemptive retellings of them.

Shifting our sense of what identity is and how it develops starts us on the path to bodyfulness, yet shaking up the identity word box isn't yet complete. We still need to question the idea that the fruition of identity lies in the mind and its largely verbally transmitted stories. Let's remember that our body tells stories as well; it shapes our identity as much as or more profoundly than words do, throughout our lifetime. We have seen that we communicate nonverbally as well as verbally. Our posture often tells an extremely accurate story about our mood and emotional state, broadcasting our emotions more effectively than words do in most cases.

Speaking with the body uses a different language system, that of movement. Movement is our first language; words come second. From tiny to large, movements operate as a signaling system to others as well as a way to talk to oneself, as we noted in chapter 5. These movements begin the process of belonging: belonging to the individual person who initiates them and the broader belonging of shared identities such as community, ethnicity, gender, and so on. We tend to repeat movements that feel right, that keep us safe, and that help us belong. We keep moving that way, and we wordlessly come to identify with the familiarity of those movements, and we begin to live by and through the fingerprint-like uniqueness of our motions. The more we move (and breathe and sense) in these ways, the more we internalize these body stories such that how we move automatically holds core features of our identity.

Because of this moving identity, our body physically holds a record of our history, called *body memory*. The way we gesture, look down as we talk, or smile at strangers all tend to reflect our history of relating to others, enacted through the body's movement habits. Are we moving through life solely from body memories, such that our bodily identity maintains itself through referencing the past? Is there room for new movements, present-moment movement experiences that will create new body stories and new bodily identities as well as recontextualize old ones? Can we take body memories under advisement rather than slavishly adhere to them? These questions can apply equally to positive and negative body memories. For instance, a positive body memory's unconscious goal might be to reinforce the behavior of sugarcoating difficult events as well as celebrating genuinely positive events. Negative body memories can help us avoid danger as well as hold us back from healing.

Body-centered psychotherapies for trauma survivors focus on these exact questions. Trauma survivors who are unresolved with their past often feel caught up in body memories that keep them jumpy, dysregulated, or numbed out in ways they can't seem to escape. Therapy often involves sensitively tracking body memories as they reemerge in present-moment treatment. For example, a tiny flexing of the wrist while talking about an attack, if brought to consciousness and allowed to tell its own story, might evolve into the hand coming up and pushing an attacker away—what the person actually wanted to do in defense during the attack, but couldn't. These conscious movement experiences, done within the current safety and relational support of therapy, can generate a new, nonverbal narration of self and identity no less important than the redemptive verbal stories the client can tell. These new body narratives empower survivors, freeing them from the grip of their body memories as the driving force of their identity.

To a lesser extent, those of us who are not trauma survivors can get stuck in our body memories in much the same way. It may be important for us to advocate for the body to tell its stories on its own terms through contemplative, expressive movement, practiced and elaborated in daily life. The body moves, and our sense of self can move and grow with it. Part of the bodyfulness construct is an ongoing dance between breathing, relating, sensing, and moving as a series of relatively autonomous "I positions"—a present-centered and quite literal positioning of the physical self in both a personal and social space. An oscillating body identity, formed by both felt and communicated movements, establishes a ground that bodyfulness can stand on and live in. Within this experience we find our empowerment.

Identity Practices

• Spontaneously write down a few words that describe your body as it is now. Notice which words might be evaluative or critical (either positive or negative). With what words would your body have been described to you by others when you were a child? How does your body respond to those words right now?

• When you have a few open minutes, try this play activity. Either by yourself or with a companion, take a minute to recall a fun experience you had. Now stand and see what it's like to retell the experience nonverbally, using only sound and body movements. The body narrative can be literal, such as mimicking eating or running, or it can be an expressionistic dance of the feeling of it, your sense of it. If you are with a companion, ask what it felt like for them to watch your moving narrative.

• If you feel up to it and have a therapist who can be with you, you may want to try this same exercise using an intense or difficult experience you have had. You can begin to physically narrate the experience more literally, but then let your body move with how it feels as it remembers the experience. It often works best if you can slow the movement down enough so that you can keep track of it and breathe with it. Stop if you lose track of your therapist, the room, or your body. Only move the experience if you can stay associated or connected to breath, sensation, movement, and relationship. Your therapist will help you keep track of this as well and guide you to stop if you can't stay in the present moment with the experience.

When the body begins to remember difficult past experiences, the practice involves attending to the experience, valuing it, and letting it complete the telling of its own story. Often, when this body story is allowed to be told through the moving body, in an atmosphere of bodyful attention and relational support, the body memory feels heard, and it can relax its grip.

The Authoritative Body

Bodyfulness follows from an *empowered* experience of self, a sense that our movements are not only understood by others but are also effective in getting our needs met and our desires fulfilled. At the simplest level, when I'm thirsty I can get up and get a glass of water. When I want to talk with someone, I can pick up the phone. When I can't do something myself, I can ask another for help. These actions are related to power. Physics defines power as the ability to do work or the rate at which work is done. As we noted before, part of the project of growing up involves learning how to use our power, our efforts, to get things done that we want or need to do. Our first and most enduring lessons about power occur through the body, as we transition in infancy from crying when we are thirsty to getting a glass of water on our own a few years later.

Some of the lessons we learn during a normal childhood involve realizing that we have to practice something as a way to get good at it and then feel powerful in our mastery of it. At the same time, we find out that we are not all-powerful, that there are limits to our power both in terms of our capabilities and in refraining from the abuse of power. Accomplishing things on our own gives us a sense of authority or authorship of our lives. We also realize that we will always need others to get some things done, and this can give us a sense of coauthorship or coauthority. Importantly, we also learn to deal with the frustration of not getting everything we want and the grief of not getting everything we need. This helps us learn the difference between authorship and dictatorship, and between acceptance and helplessness, which ideally helps us develop a healthy relationship to power. Bodyfulness revolves around how the physical self internalizes the lessons of power and authority and how bodyfulness practices can help us shake up old imprints about power and find new, more productive, and more contributive uses of it.

Bodily power and authority develop from the practice of tracking one's fluctuating physical states sensitively and seriously, and trusting one's body signals. In order to go into the kitchen and get a drink of water, I first have to pay attention to my body, read its signaling, and interpret that signal correctly as thirst. This may seem obvious, but we actually need to learn that sequence, starting in infancy. The tricky part comes when signals such as these are not in our verbal language system, telling us, for instance, to stop eating the cookies because their sweetness is spiking our blood sugar. The signal can come as a somewhat vague, heavy feeling in the belly that we have to acknowledge, interpret correctly, and take seriously. It's a bit like figuring out why a baby is crying—you guess until you get it right (and you ask other caregivers what it has meant for their babies). Parents tend to get really good at knowing exactly what their baby's cry is about, because they care so much and get a lot of practice. What if we gave that same level of caring and practice to our own body signals? Bodily authority and a right use of power grow in these somatic experiments.

As we noted before, becoming more authoritative about our body can generate a state often called *self-efficacy*. Because I'm sensitively attuned to my direct experience, I find it easier to take care of myself and to stand up for myself. When I can stand up for myself, I can more easily extend that skill to standing up for and with others. As we will discuss in the next chapter, training bodyfulness in this way may be a powerful tool in resisting oppression or injustice on both large and small scales.

All this discussion of bodily authority can take us into the tricky territory of our will—what it is and how to work with it. Will, according to the dictionary, is the means by which we decide on and initiate action, such as willing ourselves out of bed in the morning or reaching for a glass of water. It also involves deliberately controlling what we do, such as restraining the impulse to reach for one more piece of pie or biting back hurtful words. It can also mean something that is ordained, such as God's will. We tend to praise people for their willpower to resist temptations and shame people for being too willful or not having willpower. Our will can save our life or destroy it. Our will can both serve and abuse others.

Will, from the perspective of the body, involves the ability to both initiate and inhibit actions. Our neuromuscular system is actually designed along these lines. Certain brain regions, for instance, are solely devoted to planning and initiating movements, and other regions are dedicated to inhibiting and stopping movements. Brain damage in either of these regions can be devastating, resulting in an inability to connect one's will to what we physically carry out. Traumatic events, as well as childhood stress or neglect, can also create changes in these brain regions that result in movement habits that reinforce helplessness or uncontained aggression. These disturbed movement habits tend to be seen as disturbances of our will. In bodyfulness terms, our work is to consciously practice initiating and inhibiting movement so that we sharpen the skills of starting and stopping, learning when and how much to apply one or the other.

Ancient Greek philosophers, world religions, and modern-day organizations such as Alcoholics Anonymous have weighed in about our authority and will. They wisely exhort us to change the things we can, accept the things we can't change, and develop the ability to know the difference between changeable and unchangeable situations. Our body practices can help with this lifelong goal. By moving in ways that develop both effortful strength and a restful letting go of effort we create a physical base of support for our ongoing relationship to authority—ours and that of others—and our ability to discern the limits of power.

Values and ethics create an even more complex territory. Our practice of deliberately inhibiting and initiating actions, especially when connected to our conscious sensing of what we feel, helps us develop a sense of values. Moving according to our values allows us to ascertain, question, and advance our sense of ethics. I respect what I feel, and this can give me basic directions to guide my actions according to my values. Bodyful authority can also guide us in our moral development, informing us in our quest to live an ethically oriented life.

A word of caution may be in order concerning our sense of

body authority, one that can be seen occasionally on bumper stickers that exhort us to "Don't believe everything you think." Errors in thinking are common, unavoidable, and ongoing. Contemplative as well as psychotherapeutic practices help us reflect on our thinking and even challenge it at times. Psychologists often call this metacognition. At the same time, we can cultivate a *metaphysicality* of not believing everything we feel or sense bodily. Just as the mind can make errors, so can the body. It can be quiet when something is really wrong. It can send indecipherable or easily misinterpreted signals. It can crave things that are bad for it (though this is likely the result of a history of ignoring or suppressing previous correct signals, such as the nausea we felt when we smoked our first cigarette). This capacity for somatic errors may point to another fundamental difference between embodiment and bodyfulness. In embodiment we know what we feel and sense, but in bodyfulness we somatically reflect upon and even challenge our embodied experience in a way that tempers our compelling and habituated action patterns as well as our experiments with abusing power.

Powerfulness Practices

- Let's play with some weights for a minute. Wherever you are, find something that is easy to pick up, and do so, noticing the effort you use and any sense of how it feels to be able to lift that object so easily. Then find something to pick up that is challenging but doable without hurting yourself. Notice how it feels to lift that weight. What muscles do you use? How does your body shape itself around that action? How does it feel to do it? Satisfying? A bit scary? Now just play a bit with something that you have no hope of picking up (please be careful not to hurt yourself), just noticing that the effort you expend doesn't have any result. How does that feel? Frustrating? Like no big deal? Emotional? Noticing these reactions can give you clues as to your internalized relationships to your bodily authority and your relationship to power.

- Take a moment to check in with your bodily experience. Remember to just be with it for a bit, not trying to explain or rationalize your sensations. Then begin to play with your authority, hypothesizing to yourself about any problematic sensations: "This neck tension is from holding my head too far forward as I read" or "This feeling in my belly is hunger." These knowings arise because in the past you guessed correctly about what was going on, in a way that allowed you to physically solve small body problems. Do this exercise a few times, in different circumstances, and notice when you feel confident about your bodily knowing and when you feel unsure or even clueless. Often the more convinced we are of an explanation, the more suspicious of it we can be. You may want to play with both honoring and questioning your bodily authority. It might be that some persistent body problems are the result of your mis-knowing, or mis-narrating. Or it may be that a body problem needs help from others with other types of authoritative knowledge, such as health-care practitioners.

- As a wonderful variation, do the same exercise but hypothesize about pleasurable sensations.

- Take some time to slowly and deliberately play with inhibiting and initiating different movements, such as reaching, pushing, pulling, or grasping. Notice what associations come up when you do this, and acknowledge those associations as your body memories about authority, competence, will, and action.

- In order to work with your will and bodily authority, it can be useful to experiment with something tangible you struggle to resist, such as a sweet or salty food. (Don't work with something intensely toxic that you are addicted to, such as cigarettes or painkillers. You will likely need the help of others for these.) Pick a period of time—an hour, a day, or a week, for example—and engage in the following practices, in alternation:

  - Take five or so minutes, while sitting quietly, to imagine yourself *not* eating some food you tend to crave that might not be very good for you. Put in as much detail to the scene as possible.

  - Take a small portion of that food and eat it very slowly and deliberately, tracking the sensory details of the experience in as much detail as possible. This includes smelling, tasting, chewing, and swallowing. If your attention wanders, stop eating until you can bring your attention back to this food. Stop the exercise if anything about your sensory experience starts to feel negative, such as the food starts to not taste as good as you remember or you feel a bit of a bellyache. The goal of this practice is to be very conscious bodily while not eating the food, and while eating it. You may want to write down some notes about your reactions to this practice over time.

Narrating Our Bodyful Stories

How do we work with our old body stories so that we can release the grip of body memories that trap us in the past and rob us of an adaptive and principled sense of empowerment? How do we promote the construction of new body narratives that honor the past as well as serve our well-being and the well-being of others? How can we tell new body stories that engender a fluid, multiple, and permeable sense of self, where we feel not too rigidly fixed and not too disorganized or chaotic? In bodyful practice, we can know who we are, yet who we are doesn't have to be unchanging, unmalleable, or all that big of a deal. We can both trust and question our bodily authority, and we can develop a will that knows when to take a stand and when to take a seat.

The practice begins, of course, with a commitment to conscious breathing, moving, sensing, and relating. This is our base of support. Now our work is to become storytellers with our breathed, moved, sensed, and related experiences. Storytellers know that stories need to be well crafted and well delivered to be emotionally moving, comprehensible, and interesting. When these ingredients are present, stories transform us by communicating lessons, themes, values, and guidelines. Three main tasks lie before us: we must cultivate (1) the ability to tell old stories in ways that situate them as continuously helpful and meaningful, (2) the ability to generate stories in the moment that capture the essence of our present circumstances, and (3) the power to construct stories that guide us forward. Of course, we call tell these stories nonverbally, through the moving body. The key to all three tasks lies in how the body is moving right now.

WORKING WITH THE PAST

To work with specific body memories, we keep one foot in the present moment while one foot dips into the past. Before beginning, take a moment to repeat to yourself that your body memories are neither true nor untrue. Time and subsequent experiences have molded them into approximations of what actually happened; they are likely tainted by memory erosion, self-interest, and influence from others. But body memories are always meaningful. We more or less live by them, regardless of the details of what actually occurred.

We tend to repeat the imagined past because we habituate to its themes. In the body this can be quite literal—our body repeats movement sequences over and over that were constructed in the past, and the repeated sequences reinforce themselves due to energy conservation. What we repeat, we can't complete; we keep enacting our past, therefore we fail to complete our past. In the body this too can be quite literal. For instance, in the past we might have frequently cringed because we were getting hit by a bully on the playground, day in and day out. This unresolved situation causes us to choose the cringed position frequently, even into adulthood. In healthier original circumstances, we might have cringed (a sensible action), then gone to an adult who responded to the situation effectively. In the process of this resolution, our body comes back up to vertical, our breathing deepens, and our stance feels more empowered. Called *completing the movement sequence*, this resolving action constitutes a complete loop of experience—frightening event, initial defense, action to resolve, resolution, and a satisfactory release of the effort.

In bodyfulness, we don't forget the incident nor do we dramatize or minimize it. Rather, we release ourselves from being stuck in cringing. We do this by sensitively, consciously, and very deliberately completing movement sequences that empower us and help us model effective actions for those around us. Using this same playground example, we remember wanting to hit the bully to stop the attacks. As we recall the incident, we may feel our body working to organize a punch. To complete the original movement sequence, we will need to punch. However, to really empower ourselves in present circumstances, we need to refrain from setting up movement sequences that turn us into a bully, that reinforce movements that complete themselves with violence toward others. Martial arts training often resolves this dilemma through teachings that emphasize the right use of power, most notably that as we train ourselves to be capable of effective defenses such as punching, our strength will empower us not to use them.

So what do we do with the body's urge to punch back? We take it seriously but not literally. We infuse the action with bodyfulness by slowing it down, crafting it precisely, and staying awake to the details of the experience in the present moment. In this way, completing the movement sequence becomes a kind of contemplative practice rather than a reenactment of playground payback. The primary task in this practice is to move consciously while remembering, so that the present body can create a bridge from the body memory to present circumstances.

Body Memory Practice

Choose easier memories, ones less fraught with strong positive or negative valence. You should work with truly difficult memories in therapeutic circumstances, with people trained to help in this way. In this self-practice, make sure to choose some positive memories, not just difficult ones.

Take some time to remember a specific event from the past, in as much detail as possible. Now oscillate your attention between that memory and your current situation, by tracking your body while noticing your current environment. Do this oscillating until it gets easier and easier. Now, as you oscillate back to the memory, track your body there. Does the memory tend to clench your jaw, put a smile on your face, or raise your pulse? Allow the body memory sensations to develop into conscious movements. Perhaps your arm raises and your finger points, or your torso slumps, or your eyes squint. Let that happen. Just trust where your body wants to go with it. During the whole exercise, alternate your attention between the body memory and your body's presence in the room right now. The oscillations don't have to be fifty-fifty; just make sure you flow freely back and forth. Ask yourself where the movement wants to go in order to feel satisfyingly complete. Play with this completing movement with as much careful detail as possible. If it starts to feel off in any way, drop it and go back to the beginning, where the movement impulse began, and pay attention to small body signals that may be asking you to move in a different way. Just keep experimenting. If the movement starts to feel predictable, it may be best to go back again to the memory, to the point where your body started to respond to it. Trust where your body wants to go rather than where you intellectually or emotionally assume it should go. Read your sensations, particularly the ones that inform movement. The more you practice in this way, the more you will access a sense of relaxed completion at the end, and the more your body will feel free of unconsciously repeating old, unsatisfying movement strategies—and feel freer to keep choosing more satisfying ones.

When you finish with each practice time, take a moment to take stock of what happened—how your body moved and felt in the two oscillations and how the body memory motions might feel familiar in your current life. As a variation, try this exercise in the company of a friend, such that when you oscillate out, the presence of your friend as a witness can be supportive. The three goals of this exercise are to increase your capacity to move back and forth productively between body memories and current states, to be able to pair old memories to old movement patterns, and to increasingly suffuse your current, well-regulated bodily experiences into body memories, such that you move through the memories in a more empowered way.

WORKING WITH THE FUTURE

It would be truly wonderful to have the exact life we want, far into the future, all the way to the end. It might also be truly wonderful to win the lottery. As we noted before, we are in charge of some but not all of what happens to us. Many spiritual traditions ask us to stop trying so hard to get all the things we think we want, because all that wanting causes us and others to suffer. Depending on the spiritual tradition, we are asked to be grateful for what we have now, to challenge our assumption that getting what we want will make us happy, to see our lives as in the hands of God and under God's control, or to reevaluate what would actually make us truly happy. Buddhism, for instance, trains us to be as awake as possible in the present moment so as to minimize our craving for something different than *what is*, right now.

All these approaches have merit and can be used to minimize our current suffering as well as help us enter the future with grace and courage. From the perspective of the body, how do we work with what happens next—the future—all the way to our death? The answer once again lies in our movement sequencing. We just saw that to work with the past we need to resolve endings to incomplete movement sequences. In working with the future, we work with the middle of the movement sequence in order to set ourselves up for the best possible end.

Movement sequences begin when our body senses something and organizes a response to it. When we were small children, we initiated signaling movements that others, in an effort to care for us, completed for us—actions such as scooping us up and holding us as we start to get frightened. As we grew, our body got stronger and more coordinated, and our movement sequences got more complex, lengthy, and effective. These extended sequences formed the means to the ends we desired. The key to the parts of our future that we can control lies in these middle-of-the-sequence means. At times our relationship to the future feels helpless or depressing because we don't have enough practice at constructing the effective means to get there. If this disconnect with effective means happens frequently, we can lose touch with what we really feel and therefore what would really make us happy. Instead we get caught up in wanting things over which we have little control in getting. We want things—things that are meaningless or harmful to our well-being and the well-being of others—and expect the universe to magically deliver them.

Moving Toward the Future Practice

To work with our future-oriented movement sequencing, we begin with much the same instructions as the previous exercise, only now we will pay a lot more attention to the beginning of the

sequence and how to allow it to emerge and shape itself effectively.

Establish a time and place where you can play with this practice, then begin by bringing your attention inside and noticing
your bodily experience. Make sure to take time to really get a
sense of your body right now, down to subtle details. Now, attend
to something you anticipate in your future. Please don't choose
something intense such as your death or the death of a loved
one; for these big issues you should have support from others.
Keep it simple and relatively minor. Take some time to oscillate
your attention between your body here and now and the future
imagining. If this feels challenging, stop here and just keep practicing this important skill of being able to oscillate between here
and there, until the skill feels solid.

If you want to go on, start monitoring your body's responses
to the imagined future. They can be subtle, but keep attending
to them because what you pay attention to grows. As you allow
your body's responses to come into the foreground, support the
actions that want to emerge from the sensations. Let your body
move with the experience. Don't try to "get to" a desired outcome.
Let your body's motions, out of their own authority, do what they
want to do. The skill here is to inhibit movements that don't feel
connected to what your body is currently experiencing. Much like
the story about the monks counting one, two, three, four . . . and
going back to one when their mind drifted from the count, when
you find yourself moving in some expected, familiar, or habitual
way, return to the sensations that inform you of the present state
of your body. Be curious about where your body actually goes
next; it will often be in an unexpected direction.

The skill here is to gradually find the motions that feel right and support them in their exquisite detail, without making up what they mean or influencing them to a particular end. Let's say you are slowly raising your arm. Does it want to rotate ever so slightly as you raise it? Does it want to be five centimeters more forward as it goes up? Do your fingers want to curl or extend slightly? Is there an image, an emotion, a sound, a memory that comes up as you find just the right movement? Braid these associations into the action by giving them your attention; they will help you find where the movement wants to go. Stay with this experience as long as you like, oscillating your attention between your body experience, your imagined future, your associations, and your location in the present environment.

Over time, this practice will construct a kind of movement pathway, where your bodily authority can guide you toward where you want to be while at the same time showing you whether or not you really want exactly that, whether or not you are in charge of manifesting it, or whether or not the wanting of it is a smoke screen for something else. As you play with the literal movement sequences that guide you, they will over time resolve into coherent, repeatable processes that you can then experiment with applying in your daily life.

WORKING WITH THE PRESENT

Our body movement is always in the present, the past, and the future. Another way to put it is that our body is always remembering, directly experiencing, and planning—all at the same time. While from moment to moment the percentages of each may change, our brain is constantly blending all three of these standpoints to regulate itself and organize behavior. While it can be tremendously useful to separate out these three dimensions of time, the body doesn't do that. For this reason it may be useful to experiment with a fourth practice, called *movement inquiry*, which is designed to leverage present-moment experiences as a means of studying *what is*. It also establishes a stable base from which to explore the past and the future. In a way, it looks and feels a lot like sitting meditation because your instructions to stay in the present moment are the same. In many sitting meditation practices, you concentrate on one thing, such as a candle flame or mantra, or on the gap between your thoughts. In movement inquiry the object of your concentrated attention is your breathing, moving, sensing, and relating body, right now.

In this practice we pay pointed attention to our body's movement impulses and allow them to do what they want. It may or may not feel like a coherent body narrative, or a sequence with beginning, middle, and end. Your body will move with a kind of inner coherence that may transcend what you normally think of as a body story. There is no oscillating into past or future; you just keep your moving body in the present moment.[2] Another way to think about it is that working with the past and the future challenges us to move in goal-directed ways to make something happen. Our bodyfulness practice in working with the present moment challenges us to be non–goal directed in our movement to allow the present moment, as well as the past and future, to consciously happen within us.

Present Moment Movement Practice

Find a space where you can move freely and be undisturbed. Take a few minutes to check in and "warm up" by seeing what small self-care projects feel right. It may be a few stretches, some conscious breathing, or foot rubbing. When you feel ready, let your body get as quiet as possible, and attend to the details of what is happening both inside and outside your body. Your eyes can open or close all through this practice—do what feels right in the moment. Throughout the practice, work to gently bring your attention back to your embodied experience whenever it wanders. Pay special attention to small movements in your body, perhaps your heartbeat or your breathing. You can just stay with that or you can extend the practice to more observable motions.

When we attend to the body in its present state, without judgment, analysis, or the expectation that it needs to move a certain way, the body often brings up movement on its own. It may be that your arm wants to rise up, your head wants to tip, or your spine wants to curl over. Trust what seems to want to happen. If you notice yourself manufacturing movements out of habit, note that and come back to the quietness of your breath and your heartbeat. There is no place the body needs to go, yet it can go wherever the wind of focused attention takes it. The movements that show up tend to be slow, but this isn't required. Let your body, via its own authority, choose its speed and the amount of space it takes up. Making sounds can be part of the movement.

Conclude the practice when it feels right, though it may be best to initially plan to spend about ten minutes and work up to twenty or thirty minutes when it feels right. When you feel finished, take some time to do any self-care activities, as you did in the beginning. You may want to write down what you noticed during your movement time.

In a sense, we want our whole life to be a satisfyingly completed movement sequence, from conception to death, where we can feel complete when things end. While we don't have control over all our endings, this resting into the authority of our awakened and moving body may be one of our most powerful ways to find more satisfaction with endings. We can move in ways that construct body stories that identify us and feel coherent. We can also move in ways that deconstruct our past and future narratives in the crucible of the present moment so that new identities and new authorities may emerge. An oscillation ensues that empowers our dreams and remembrances as well as empowers us to experience ourselves, right now. We experience our aliveness and awakened presence in all locations on this continuum. For some spiritual paths, the cultivation of enlightenment involves an ongoing state of occupying the present moment. In bodyfulness, we acknowledge the physical realities and presence of the past and the future in our body as it occupies the present moment. Because of this, we neither worship the present moment nor avoid it but rather see the present moment as the extensive middle ground of our awakened oscillations.

8

Bodylessness and the Reclamation of Bodily Authority

THE PREVIOUS CHAPTER positioned us within practices that cultivate our bodyful stories and our bodyful authority. Now it's time to flip this word box called *bodyfulness* over and ask ourselves how a state of *bodylessness* could also exist, what it looks like, and what we should do about it. We can see this new word *bodylessness* as holding four conditions: (1) ignoring the body, (2) seeing the body as an object or project, (3) hating the body, and (4) making one's own or other people's bodies wrong. The result of bodylessness is a life lived at a distance from who we were, who we are, and who we will be. This distance from ourselves causes us to suffer more, feel less pleasure, treat others poorly, and experience more challenges in living a self-reflective life.

Ignoring the Body

One of the ways we can understand junk food, smoking, ongoing binge watching, drug abuse, and other addictions is by noticing that they all get started and are maintained by repeatedly ignoring or minimizing our body's signals and actions, such as the nausea, headache, and loss of coordination that show up as we start to practice them. Research shows that many of us tend to be aware of our body only under three conditions: sex, exercise, and pain. While attending to the body during these states is laudable, it's not nearly enough to be embodied, much less bodyful. Turning our attention away from our body can at times be useful; an example would be during the physical pain associated with an illness or injury that we have addressed as much as we can and must simply wait for it to pass, in which case it might be just fine to read a book or take an aspirin. But both embodiment and bodyfulness require that we unconditionally oscillate our attention into our body as well as away from it on an ongoing and contemplative basis.

Research shows that we can cultivate increased sensory acuity with practice—whether that be our sense of smell, taste, touch, or interoception—simply by paying more focused attention to these senses more frequently. We can also gain motor skills, particularly proprioception and kinesthesia, through conscious movement practices that require us to use them repeatedly. Bodylessness turns away from these conscious practices in an attempt to ignore the body messages that might come as a result. There are three main reasons we ignore our body: pain avoidance, cultural pressure, and mistaking obliviousness for rest.

If, historically, our physical or emotional pain was too intense, too unrelenting, or too often outside our control, we likely have set up habits that keep our attention elsewhere. As well, the various cultures we live in—our family, community, ethnicity, religion, and institutions such as schools and governments—have had their own historical reasons for ignoring the body, and as a result they will pressure us to do the same, calling it tradition, ritual, laws, or policies. Sometimes these codes are written, and sometimes unwritten.

If, historically, we have worked too hard at something too many times and for too long, we habituate to ignoring body signals that urge us to rest or to do something different, such as play. It can be important to push ourselves like this occasionally, such as walking that last mile down a street, even though our feet hurt, in order to get home. But a consistent practice of ignoring our felt experience will set up the habit of ignoring body signals during work and collapsing at the end of work in exhaustion. Instead of an ongoing and satisfying alternation of work, rest, and play, we get sucked into a sequence of work, work, collapse. The overwork comes with obvious costs, yet so does the collapse, which often involves oblivious activities such as hours and hours on the couch, in front of a device, or on a barstool.

Seeing the Body as an Object or Project

We can ignore our body, and we can also distort it when we do attend to it. Two terms describe how we can distort our bodily selves: *body as object* and *body as project*. We often see our body as a thing that "we," a mental self, live inside of—much like a vessel or a machine. While we might be good at maintaining this vessel or machine, treating the body as an object is the first step in objectifying ourselves and others. When our body becomes an object, it loses rights, dignity, compassion, authority, and bodyfulness.

A version of this objectification occurs when we take on our body as a project, most often as an improvement project. When our body deviates from an idealized norm, we go to the gym, the plastic surgeon, or the cosmetics counter. We consult social media for guidance in how we should appear. We don't see our body as good enough the way it is, and we evaluate ourselves and others on the authority of fashion designers, commercials, and popular magazines, frequently without even realizing we are doing it. When we commoditize our physical form in this way, we push our appearance into the foreground and our lived experience into background. Our bodily self is then driven by consumer culture, and our inclusion or exclusion in social circles can depend on how often we work out, how many beauty products we buy, and how well we disguise physical "flaws" and the aging process. We stage our body rather than celebrate it, look at it rather than feel it.

Certainly taking care of our physical health and appearance carries with it all sorts of important benefits, many of which are bound up in a bodyful life. But when we treat our body as a thing, we lock in a kind of self-aggression, ignorance, and persecution of ourselves and others that exacts a toll. In consumerist-based economies, profits depend on companies conning us into thinking that wrinkles mean failure, aging is appalling, and being gendered has certain strict rules of dress and comportment. Racist, sexist, and homophobic groups capitalize on our tendency to objectify ourselves and con us into treating bodies different from our own, however unconsciously, as foreign objects to be feared and marginalized.

Hating the Body

All this builds up to hating the body, what we called *somatophobia* earlier in the book. When we accuse our bodily self of being ugly, wrong, stupid, or slow, we set ourselves up for psychological distress and self-harm. Several common erroneous assumptions fuel this distress.

The first error has to do with how we handle our fear of illness and death. It's difficult for us to accept our death and relatively easy to hope that some noncorporeal self will not get sick or die. Since the body obviously doesn't persist past death, perhaps there is some nonmaterial essence of us that does. In many cultures we call this our *soul*. But for the soul to persist past death, it has to break bonds with the impermanent body. If we think that will happen at our death, it can be an easy extension to assume that separateness exists before our death, as there from the start. This separation can lead to arbitrary distinctions between body and soul that push the body into the landscape of "wrong."

The second error centers around pain. Even though we can experience persistent and intense psychological or emotional pain, physical pain can often overwhelm us in such powerful ways that it can be hard to express in words. It can be difficult not to blame our body for this, for doing something wrong or for being weak, fragile, or faulty. It's also easy to assume that there is a separate and more ideal part of us that doesn't feel that pain. A related version of this error reveals itself when we state that "the spirit is willing, but the flesh is weak," meaning that the corporeal self succumbs to wrongdoing but our higher self would never do such things.

Our third error concerns the body's vulnerability to being controlled. People can imprison or constrain our body, but we can sit in that jail and think what we want. Our mind is relatively free, and this small blessing and important escape can lead us to the idea that our body is simpler and more problematic. The part of us we call our mind can go anywhere, into flights of imagination, fun fantasies, and dissociative escapes from suffering. In our imaginings, we can fly, do magic, and construct the exact retort that would have put that person in their place. In the abstract, we are not limited by the physics, chemistry, and biology of the body. However, if we consistently mentalize as an escape from being physically controlled or limited in some way, we can set up an assumption that our physicality is the problem. Once we separate our ability to abstract from our ability to enact, we blame our body for being dumber, plodding, and uncreative.

One of the most threatening things Charles Darwin did when he posited natural selection as a force that operated on all life-forms was when he deduced that humans are a type of animal. This brings us to another all too common illusion of separateness. This dethroning of humans as wholly separate from and superior to other animals has been upsetting to many, to say the least. The more we identify with our body, the more we have to come to grips with our animal nature, and we typically equate "animal nature" with primitiveness, soullessness, immorality, and stupidity. Darwin's denial of humans as a separate and "better" life-form, coupled with his unifying of all life-forms into a kind of diverse family, is so rattling that in the United States 42 percent of us still refuse to believe that it's true.[1] This refusal can also lead us to a related error, that of seeing the body as the lowly animal part of our nature and the mind or the soul as the elevated, separate, nonanimal part of our identity. Again, somatophobia, a mild to acute hatred of the body, rests on a core assumption of separateness.

Somatophobia is internalized as self-criticism of one's own body and externalized by critiquing others' bodies. (Do an Internet search for "body troll," an online body bullying phenomenon.) It's both implicit (operating below conscious awareness) and explicit (consciously enacted). It's a costly error to individuals, groups, and communities and gets echoed and repeated on a systems level when our bodily authority is subjugated to the state, the church, or the school.

The bias we absorb and enact can poison our inner experience and be communicated to others as well. Research shows that bias is contagious, infecting whole communities and normalizing hatefulness toward others. It can be wholly learned implicitly and can therefore be denied. This same research shows that bias is often communicated through nonverbal behaviors.[2] Clearly we need to be responsible to and for our own body while at the same time appreciating and being responsible for what our body communicates to others. By using bodyful practices to surface internalized body biases, we not only serve ourselves but also learn to consciously refrain from *othering* people different than ourselves.

Making Specific Bodies Wrong

One of the first ways an individual or group can oppress another is to make their body wrong—the wrong color, size, shape, posture, gesture, or movement. Social theory literature sometimes calls this *othering*. How do we not only make bodies in general inherently less valuable than the mind but also *other* specific bodies that are different from our own in such a way that oppression and social injustice ensue? What are the effects of this oppression in the bodies of the people who are marginalized for being somatically different?

Making particular bodies wrong, which I will call *somaticism*, involves targeting the physical culture of a group as well as doing violence to their bodies, whether enacted through ethnicity, race, gender, ability, size, age, or socioeconomic status. In this type of oppression, specific body parts, postures, gestures, movements, use of space, eye contact, voice tone, body size, body shape, and other markers of the body are singled out as evidence of being a member of a nondominant group, and that evidence is used to lower status and physical safety, diminish rights, and exclude the *othered* from resources. For instance, when the norm is a thin, young, fit, light-skinned, symmetrical body—clearly marked as male or female—that moves the way the dominant group moves, then anyone who doesn't fall into those categories will experience some kind of exclusion. This exclusion typically rounds up and segregates people of color, the disabled, the young, the poor, and the gender noncon-forming. In some cases, this exclusion costs certain people their lives, either through violence, relentless stress, or self-harm. Some of the less lethal and ongoing results of this exclusion likely involve a lifetime of self-criticism, work to control one's body appearance and activities, chronic health issues, projecting one's "deficiencies" onto others, and exhausting attempts to either fit in or resist the dominant body narrative.

Indeed, the concept of embodiment itself may be contaminated by white privilege. A colleague of mine, Carla Sherrell, has written about "titrated embodiment," noting that as an African American woman moving in white culture, it is often not safe for her to be embodied, as this would be too threatening to those around her. Instead, she chooses to go in to and out of embodiment so that she can navigate racism effectively. Another colleague, Beit Gorski, a trans and genderqueer activist and therapist, writes about the value and importance of dissociation as a strategy to cope with discrimination and as a way to challenge our narrow and often oppressive ideas about mental health.[3]

The Cultured Body and Difference

Our body is an enculturated creature, and it's through studying culture that we can identify the flip side of the separation errors listed above and expose the opposite error to which we often fall prey: the need to think things are as similar as possible. How different can our body culture get from another's before we make either their body or ours wrong? For some, the distance should be minimal—"others" should assimilate, accommodate, and do their utmost to blend in with "us." For others, it may be too permissive, such that we give certain cultural practices (such as torture) a pass when we shouldn't. In this scenario, we manage our fear of difference by denying that some differences are not okay. In both cases, the politics of cultural difference lands with a violent thud on the body. We tend to fear difference and seek to reduce it, requiring others to move, dress, and behave as we do. Regardless of how we cope, this fear lurks below conscious awareness, causing us to deny that we carry bias.[4]

Like the individual body, cultures can be mapped along multiple continuums as well. One of the most salient measures is the continuum from individualism and collectivism. From a body perspective, an individualistic culture sees the body as separate, on its own, and self-determined. In collectivistic cultures, the body is seen as related to, affected by, and connected to other bodies, whether that be those of ancestors or kin. The bodily self is more a group self. Highly individualistic cultures tend to be located in Scandinavia, Western Europe, and North America. Collectivistic cultures tend to be in Central and South America, Africa, and Asia. The frequency of touching also maps onto this continuum, as low-touch cultures tend to be more individualistic, and high-touch cultures tend to be more collectivistic. The same is true for the use of space: collectivistic cultures tend to require less space around the body when interacting with others than individualistic cultures. What happens in us when we encounter the body of someone who occupies a different place on this cultural continuum than we do?

Cultures also map onto continuums regarding authority, resulting in relatively flat to relatively tiered social hierarchies in which body gestures, postures, dress, use of space, and voice tone are used to nonverbally communicate status in the hierarchy. All cultures also create notions about gender and how fluid or rigid gender designations and roles should be. These notions about gender can be slightly to highly constraining of the body, affecting how it sits, faces, gestures, and positions itself in space so as to signal gender identity and create safety in gendered spaces.

Our human tendency to measure the body on cultural continuums helps us play with and play out themes of sameness and difference, separation and unity, tolerance and intolerance. How we work with these themes also pulls in our relationship to bodyfulness and bodylessness. In states of bodylessness, we disembody (ignore) ourselves and others, we mis-embody ourselves and others (body as object), we feel somatophobic (hatred) toward ourselves and others, or we feel critical of body difference (somaticistic) of ourselves and others. Bodyfulness now becomes an active force that can bring us back from this hurtful and hurting place.

Bodyfulness as Activism

Making the body "less than" and making specific, different bodies into the "other" are categories that almost always overlap, creating a double whammy for nondominant individuals and groups. Both categories create popular narratives that construct and maintain the marginalization of the body, narratives that are unexamined rationalizations at best. At their worst, these narratives delegitimize our body and the bodies of others and legitimize the oppression and violence enacted as a result.

Perhaps the cultivation of bodyfulness on a social level can be one way to vaccinate ourselves against social injustice and autocracy. If individual members of a society learned to readily know and value what they feel, if they listened to and respected their embodied experience, they might be more equipped to resist being "othered" and less likely to succumb to any social pressure to "other" people different than themselves. A person who keeps track of their embodied experience is more likely to keep track of their rights as an embodied being, value the rights of others, and feel empowered enough to stand up for them effectively. This idea guides us to an even deeper understanding of the body's relationship to power. As Martin Luther King Jr. said in his 1967 sermon at the 11th Annual Southern Christian Leadership Conference, "Power properly understood is nothing but the ability to achieve purpose. It's the strength required to bring about social, political, and economic change."[5]

At this point, we may be willing to contemplate the idea that our body is our own as well as bound up with others and that part of the reason we empower our body is to use that power in the service of others, most notably those in need. This idea pervades most world religions, for good reason. It also pervades bodyfulness in the form of bodyful activism. What this activism looks like for each of us is up to us to decide. What it will involve is feeling our body's power and acting on it by moving, breathing, sensing, and relating in the service of our own and others' rights. This activism, according to Dr. King, involves love. In the same sermon mentioned above, he stated that "power at its best is love implementing the demands of justice, and justice at its best is love correcting everything that stands against love. And this is what we must see as we move on."[6]

Bodyful activism begins with loving our body. But it doesn't stay there, otherwise love, according to Dr. King, becomes "anemic and sentimental."[7] It claims a kind of inner justice so that our internalized bodily ignorance, our sense of physical wrongness, and our sense of fusion or separation can fade. As our inner experience of justice grows, our outer actions have an experiential template from which to make use of our power, together, for all of us.

Chapter Practices

- If you are up for it, take out a piece of paper and write down ten or so adjectives about your body—one-word descriptors that come to mind, without censoring. Look over the list. Which words have positive connotations and which have negative connotations? Could any of them be somatophobic? Just notice what comes up as you acknowledge that you used these words.

- If you are feeling brave, you can do this same writing exercise focused on someone else's body, preferably one that is quite different from your own. It could be a close friend or a stranger. Look at the list. How many of the words are evaluative? Could any of them be somatophobic? How does the second list compare to the first list? Don't overthink it; just feel the details of the experience you are having as you do the exercise. Almost all of us routinely make bodies wrong, whether it be for size, shape, age, ability, or ethnicity. These exercises are not designed to be "gotcha" experiences. In either of these exercises, if you notice shame or guilt, for instance, you are not yet at a truly self-reflective place. Shame and guilt almost always cover over more important feelings and obscure the more bodyful feelings of personal responsibility and even remorse. If you notice guilt or shame, try labeling them as another manifestation, another layer, of your somatophobia or somaticism.

- The path to loving your body and others' bodies the way they are is to sense, breathe, move, and relate to them. Begin by identifying internalized bodylessness, as we started to do in the exercises above. As you get more comfortable with identifying your moments of bodylessness (as they manifest in words, actions, thoughts, and feelings), you may want to move with and sequence that experience so that you can complete body memories that may have set them up. When you get a palpable sense of how bodylessness feels, you are already starting to dissolve it. The sequencing goes like this: (1) identify the details of the bodylessness, (2) reframe any shame or wrongness as the feeling component of the bodylessness, (3) stay with your body, attending to any sensations, associations, or movement impulses that form, (4) allow body stories to emerge and allow them to sequence. If none emerge, go back to the beginning of the sequence; no worries. Don't be surprised if this becomes a frequent and long-term practice.

- Take a few minutes to locate yourself on the individualistic/ collectivistic cultural continuum. It may be a bit different now than when you were growing up. Reflect for a bit on what it has been like to interact with others who are in similar or different locations on the continuum, particularly how your body responded to their bodies. Recall the physical details of these experiences. Was the interaction memorable because of use of space, appearance, movement style, touch? Working with cultural differences isn't easy. Use body awareness to identify the somatic details of what you really feel when interacting with others, whether it be curiosity, repulsion, pity, or attraction. Apply the same sequence as in the exercise above.

- As a variation of this exercise, look at and work with your body and the bodies of others through the lenses of gender, ability, race, socioeconomic status, and color.

9

When Being Here Takes You There

Change and the Body

AFTER CONTEMPLATING OUR identity from a bodyful location, a related question having to do with the nature of change emerges. Identity can be seen as a feature of our stability, and change can be seen as our source of mobility. Bodyfulness lies in our conscious oscillation between these two features of movement. Whether it's changing our minds, our hearts, or our habits, we all can struggle with when, how, and whether to stay put or go somewhere else. We often strive to be in control of change, wanting to be change agents rather than at the mercy of other people, systems, or fate. Yet we tend to find it difficult to change in many cases, knowing we should stop a bad habit, for instance, but not doing so. Why do we want (or not want) to change, where does the desire to change come from, and how do we accomplish it?

One way we can begin to sort out these questions is to see change as often complex and involving conflicting forces; it doesn't necessarily arise from a single source or from a clear sense of direction. We also know that change is constant, it can be planned or unplanned, it can be devastating or exhilarating. One definition for *change* in the dictionary is "the absence of monotony." Since we know that both the physical body and the state of bodyfulness seek to avoid excessive monotony, let's look through a somatic lens to understand where change comes from, where our motivation to change comes from, and how we can work with change bodyfully.

Where Change Comes From

Once again, let's put this topic on a continuum. At one extreme change comes entirely from outside of us (an external locus of control). Something shifts in a way that lies completely outside of our will, abilities, or power. In the broad middle ground of the continuum lies our ability to influence change, where we have varying percentages of power to steer the process. At the other extreme, changes lie completely within our abilities (an internal locus of control). To put it succinctly, some change comes from elsewhere and happens to us, a lot of change is under some degree of our influence, and some change comes entirely from within. As we noted before, our bodyfulness practice permits us to locate our current experience along this continuum with increasing amounts of accuracy, so that we can act wisely.

Change that happens to us from outside forces can be a mixed bag. On one hand, it can be a relief to just let ourselves be transformed by someone or something else, as long as it's perceived as beneficial. Winning the lottery falls into this category. But the key ingredient is that we are not in charge of the change—we may feel lucky or unlucky, but we don't feel powerful. On the other hand, this kind of change can come in the form of tragedy. An example of this occurred in my private practice many years ago, when I was counseling a seventeen-year-old young man who was struggling with his relationship to his father. In the midst of our work together, his father was suddenly killed in a car accident. My client's world abruptly and traumatically broke apart and would never be the same. Not only did he lose his father, but he had to move out of his house and change schools. Part of his shock and grief took him in the direction of incorrectly assuming that because he had been angry with his father he had somehow caused his death. Our sessions alternated between working directly with his raw and overwhelming emotions and gently but inexorably exerting pressure on his error about where this change had come from. When both these states gradually stabilized over the next months, we were able to shift toward working with his present circumstances and his altered course into the future. Accurately identifying when change isn't invited or influenceable can help us ride the experience instead of be swept away by it.

If change happens to us and there is nothing we can do to prevent or shape it, our wise responses tend to move us toward acceptance and active accommodation. We can reduce our suffering by changing our relationship to circumstances that we can't change. For instance, in the field of psychology, we are seeing mindfulness and acceptance-based therapies emerge, techniques that cultivate a relaxed, nonadversarial relationship to one's current state, where upsetting sensations, emotions, and thoughts are allowed to come and go.[1] These therapies are amassing impressive results, particularly with clients who are experiencing unavoidable suffering (such as chronic pain). The danger here lies in the distinction between acceptance and passivity. By staying active with one's states and by experimenting with the possibilities of influencing one's situation as well as accepting it, we develop the skill of oscillating skillfully along the change continuum.

People who live in poverty, who live in war zones, or who face discrimination and marginalization experience more of this change-from-the-outside than others. Such change often results in a sense of powerlessness and hopelessness that can be quite crippling and often transgenerational. In these cases, acceptance and accommodation look very different. What an oppressive system wants is for the bodies of the people it targets to feel this powerlessness, to believe that they are the cause of it, and to shut up and accept it. The bodyfulness practice in these circumstances initially entails accepting that they didn't do anything to cause this trauma to happen, much like my client above. What has happened to these people, and what continues to happen to them, comes from elsewhere. The accommodation involves learning to physically work with the situation as it is now and empower themselves and others to bodyfully push back against the systems that create these conditions.

When change processes come from inside us, we initiate them from our own feelings and interests. No outside force impels us to do anything different, yet we feel an inner urge to shift. In this condition our task is to bodyfully initiate, sequence, and complete the change process using our inner dictates to craft the change that feels right. As we saw in the previous chapter, the practice that matches this change experience involves movement inquiry. By not willing our body to move in one direction or the other, we find new directions that feel right, that organize themselves from present-moment experiences rather than automatically repeating old habits. For those of us who have and are experiencing trauma or oppression, this practice can be a powerful experience of finding the body we are rather than the body we were told to have.

Another way to look at self-initiated change invokes our top-down/bottom-up principle. Top-down change uses cognitive and mental processes to alter our actions—a kind of trickle-down economics that forms the basis of insight-based practices. If we change our thinking, if we understand ourselves more deeply, we can influence our behavior. Bottom-up change arises from our body and holds to the idea that we have to shift our physical state and our behavior in order to turn things around. Behaviorally, we learn to calm ourselves down, count to ten before speaking, breathe deeply, not reach for the drink, and learn to make better eye contact, for instance. Ideally, a bodyful practitioner knows how to value and use both these directions of self-initiated change. Using only one or the other can unbalance our experience of change.

In the middle of our change continuum lies the extensive terrain of a mix of inside and outside influences impelling change. The complexity of learning to locate oneself in this mix involves a lifelong practice of combining acceptance and accommodation with initiating, sequencing, and completing movement processes in ways that honor the amount of influence we have over the course of our lives. An example would be our health. If we look at cancer, for instance, we can see that some cancers come from outside us, such as from radiation from a nuclear reactor meltdown. Others are largely self-inflicted, such as contracting lung cancer after years of smoking. Most cancers carry a mix of influences: lifestyle behaviors, genetics, environmental contaminants, avoidable and unavoidable stressors. Pragmatically, our job is to identify the portions of our cancer risk we have control over—diet, physical activity, and other lifestyle factors—and conscientiously influence our cancer risk as much as we can, using both top-down and bottom-up strategies. As well, we can contribute to collective change by actively pushing back against carcinogenic pollutants or by supporting cancer research. From a bodyfulness perspective, our work is to oscillate bodily effort and the release of effort to help us find the current percentage of influence we have over the change process.

Part of this mix of influences includes our assessment of how much we can do on our own and how much we need help from other people or things. For instance, if we feel depressed, we can call a friend, engage in more social contact, or challenge ourselves to get more exercise.[2] After trying these strategies and doing what we can, we might still need the help of antidepressant medications, and/or we may need to make bigger changes, such as changing jobs or ending a relationship. In cases of trauma, injustice, or oppression, resting into the support and collective actions of and with others can accomplish change more effectively and less stressfully than individual action. It all boils down to whether the change is larger than we are; whether it overwhelms our current identity or our resources. If we can do something about our change on our own, we feel basically empowered and affirmed. When we can't do anything about change, we can access humility and equanimity. Grace commences in either of those bodyful locations. In the broad middle ground our grace shows up in the continuous dance of moving with the exquisite details of the different influences, individually and collectively.

Motivations for Change

What gives us the energy to change? Physics tells us that any change of state requires an input of energy. How do we get the energy for the destabilizing work of changing the status quo, either within ourselves or in the outer world? We get our energy from three possible sources: being pushed, seeking pleasure, and being curious.

Charles Darwin and Alfred Wallace have taught us about the phenomenon of being pushed to change. Their discovery of the laws of natural selection starts from the observation that life-forms don't change unless they need to. Since life-forms seek to conserve energy to survive and thrive, evolution will not occur unless the environment changes, and who we currently are and how we currently do things no longer enable us to survive and thrive. Either we change, or we go extinct. Being pushed into change means we don't choose it, and we often object to it and resist it.

The force that pushes us feels like pressure from the outside— pressure from family to stop drinking, pressure from relationship breakups to question our relational skills, pressure to go on living after a child dies. In some cases, this pressure, though unanticipated and often unwelcome, is quite natural, such as pressure from the death of an aged loved one, illness, or our own aging. In other cases, the pressure rises from others because we are not making needed changes on our own. This could involve our loved ones getting fed up with our self-destructive habits or the court system informing us that if we get one more DUI we will go to jail. We are forced into change, in many cases unwillingly.

The "pressure" symptoms can be physical, such as headaches that show up as we drive to work. They can be expressed through emotions—such as feeling pushed around and overwhelmed by fear or sadness. They can be cognitive, showing up as projections or rationalizations that are off the mark. Or they can be social or relational, playing out in an unhappy relationship or a lack of friends. Pressured change usually finds its root in themes of survival, safety, and functionality, and this can be why we sometimes resist change—staying the same feels as if our life or our identity depends on it. As in cases of prolonged stress, we sometimes simply don't have the spare energy to effect change.

We all experience change in this way, even the most enlightened among us. There is no getting around painful, pressured changes, though we can certainly live in ways that minimize them and lessen the struggle and suffering we experience because of them. Bodyful change in response to pressure often starts out as not wanting to hurt so much. It can be tempting to simply sedate the message with distractions, denial, or drugs. Ultimately bodyfulness teaches us to identify, respect, and address pain signals. The practices we will work with in the next section emphasize listening to the signals and giving them a voice. By doing this, we can more accurately and bodyfully respond to what the messages are telling us, as well as form a healthier relationship to pain in which we work with it to solve problems and change things.

Our second motivation to change is simply and elegantly expressed by the Dalai Lama, who notes that we all want to be happy—we all have that in common. We possess a natural inclination to go toward things that please us and that help us feel better. This inclination may explain our playfulness as a species and our ability to leverage play as a change agent. While pressure-based change works by using various painful symptoms as a means of motivating us to change, pleasure-based change works through positive states. Feeling pleasure as a result of our own actions—whether it be laughing at a joke, enjoying a sunset, having contactful sex, or dancing to music—carries all kinds of physical, emotional, and cognitive health benefits. The key to these benefits, and to making changes because of them, lies in developing a healthy relationship to pleasure.

One way to talk about a healthy relationship to pleasure is to make a distinction between *active pleasures* and *passive pleasures*. Active pleasures, as noted above, entail experiences where we generate pleasure via something we do. We move in some certain way in order to feel better, happier. This solidifies the connection between our purposeful moving and our positive feelings, increasing our sense of self-efficacy and empowerment. Active pleasures don't need to be physically demanding; they can include a deeply active listening to music, for instance, because it takes energy to really listen.

In passive pleasures we remain receptive to the positive feeling, but we don't work to produce it. It just happens to us. Passive pleasures sometimes involve experiences where pleasure is in some way forced upon us, such as drinking alcohol or taking drugs. Basically when we ingest substances such as these, they work in our brain by forcing pleasure centers to stay more stimulated for longer than we can typically produce ourselves through our own actions. While pleasures such as these can be fun and entertaining, they don't produce lasting benefits or change. In cases where we choose passive methods of feeling pleasure consistently and excessively, habituation and addiction can result because the brain mechanisms cited above become exhausted and less sensitive to self-directed pleasure. They don't make us happier, and in many cases they can make us much more unhappy.

In cases such as excessively strict parenting, chronic stress, marginalization, or simply enduring a humorless childhood, we can habituate to experiencing a low limit of pleasure. When life comes along and presents us with something truly joyful, we can feel anxious and threatened. Part of the job of a happy childhood is to learn to tolerate and produce active pleasures. Part of the job of bodyfulness is to practice and get used to everyday, natural, and normal enjoyments. By reaching out actively to feel better, in very conscious and conscientious ways, we change for the better.

Play, particularly physical play, can be an important strategy in the development of our pleasure abilities. As adults, our play can be more inclusive and complex than for children. Even though it can work wonderfully to play with kids and like a kid, we adults need a larger repertoire. If we again define play as anything we do for the sole purpose of doing it, adult play can include such activities as chess, sex, and even spiritual practices. Doing these things bodyfully can generate powerful, wanted, and lasting change in our lives.

Our third and last motivation to change takes us away from the realms of pain and pleasure, where we learn to work effectively with urges to move away from or toward things. In our third motivation, called *inquiry*, we learn to work with an urge to "move with," as well as to work with, no urges at all. Whether an experience is painful or pleasurable loses its relevance. In this method of change, we expend our energy in the service of active responsiveness to the present moment. While working with pain and pleasure can be said to be goal-oriented activities (having an outcome in mind), working with inquiry helps us understand how to get better at non-goal-oriented states and, paradoxically, to leverage them toward change. We simply rest into what is and then pair it with how we are moved as a result. One way to understand inquiry is to use a movement metaphor. As we saw before, movement involves an oscillation between expending effort and releasing effort. Pressure and pleasure, because of their inherent urgings to move us toward or away from things, require effort to guide change. In inquiry, we let go of effort because we are already there. Our sense of empowerment and self-efficacy arises from a deep immersion in the body as it acts, right here and now.

Another way to understand change through inquiry is to dip into the literature on creativity. One of our best means of doing that is to investigate the concept of *flow*.[3] Flow describes the state one is in while being creative, and it shares some interesting characteristics with bodyfulness, and particularly with inquiry. In flow, our awareness merges with our actions. It's a state of "self-forgetfulness," where we are also very awake and very absorbed in the present moment. To enter flow we need to sharpen our attention to the task at hand and practice actions that slightly test our ability. To cultivate flow states, we work to oscillate along multiple continuums as the occasion requires. These continuums include: playful to disciplined, detached to attached, imaginative to reality orientated, extroversion to introversion, humility to pride, and rebelliousness to conservativism.

Remember that in several stages of life our brain overproduces neurons, and the ones that don't get used die off. These are times where change becomes much more likely. By entering the flow states connected with inquiry, especially movement inquiry, we likely can grow and sustain new neural pathways that allow our brain-body to be more and more creative, not only for artistic purposes but also within daily living.

This brings us to the idea that being here can take you there. Pressure, pleasure, and inquiry all contain paradoxes. Change paradoxically seems to require that we acknowledge, befriend, and engage with the way things are, here and now, before they can go anywhere else. The way things are is our home base. In 1996 Sylvia Boorstein wrote a meditation book called *Don't Just Do Something, Sit There*. This delightful title pushed back on our old adage of "don't just sit there, do something." Yet if we throw either one away and just value the other, we miss the wonderful oscillation between life's goal-oriented and non-goal-oriented moments. Whenever we move, we are always moving toward something and away from something else. The answer to change doesn't involve stopping our motion altogether so that we eliminate attraction or repulsion. The answer lies in moving bodifully in all directions. Life requires that we know how to just sit there and also how to get up and move toward and away from things. Bodyfulness imbues each of these three activities when we start with nonjudgmentally sensing, moving, breathing, and relating with where we are right now. This known location creates a map around us that illuminates our path when changing our location becomes necessary, advisable, or of interest.

We can see that a recurring theme in this section has to do with active engagement during change processes, whether it be with pressures, pleasures, or inquiries. This activeness keeps us in optimal territory for change to be positive. This truism came home to me many years ago when I was learning to white-water canoe. After learning the different paddle strokes and principles, we went through some small rapids. I worked very, very hard, using my paddle and my will to control precisely where the canoe should go. The problem was that this didn't work, and I ended up dunked, my canoe going downstream without me. I tried again, working even harder, and got dunked again. It was exhausting and irritating, so I decided that I had been too controlling (duh) and that I should let go and literally go with the flow. I ran the rapids again, just letting the waves and currents take me where they would, but with the same result—me in the river, the empty canoe going downriver without me. After a second failed attempt at going with the flow,

I had the good sense to watch my instructor navigate these cursed rapids. He went through with utmost grace. He didn't paddle constantly, but when he did use a stroke, it was timed and executed in ways that cooperated with what the water was doing while at the same time leveraging it to position himself in the flow in ways that got him downstream, relatively dry and inside his canoe. What really struck me was that he was having fun while I had been miserable.

Negative change will always happen. Even advanced canoers occasionally take a swim, and some rapids are just too wild to be canoed safely. What active engagement teaches us is that we can work with the change process in ways that lessen the likelihood of suffering and increase the likelihood of satisfying outcomes. This "working with" skill develops when we pay high-quality attention to the river and to our place in it, and when we relate our body to the body of the canoe and to the body of the river. We are connected, and by experiencing this connection and paddling with it, we often come through with a sense of satisfying completion and a deeper understanding of ourselves and the world.

We often resist change because we haven't had enough experiences like this. We have been taught to avoid rivers, or we have had terrible experiences on them (such as a lack of instruction or being thrown into raging torrents). To change metaphors and use a more psychological lens, we could say that when we don't have enough physical, emotional, or cognitive resources, we can't experience our connection to change events. We can't stay associated to the events, and the result is dissociation. In a dissociated state, we become quickly overwhelmed and can't actively engage with them. In this scenario negative outcomes will be all too common, while positive outcomes will only be through chance. The reason that breathing, moving, sensing, and relating form the core principles of bodyfulness is because they keep us associated to our experiences and they teach us how to get better at more and more challenging change experiences.

Advanced Change—Novelty

Oscillating between doing something and sitting there, what we are calling active engagement, can help us learn to work with change. We start this practice by identifying and appreciating the details of our present state, and by themselves these skills can help immensely with many change processes. What grows from these root skills of identifying and appreciating can be just as useful, and that is the ability to work with novelty. Remember how change can be defined as the absence of monotony? In the absence of monotony, novelty emerges. Novelty is what we experience when we move into a new state, one that exists outside habit and automaticity. While we know that habit and automaticity are crucial to our survival and happiness, they don't work unless they alternate with the unplanned, unbidden, and unexplored. Creative processes emerge from these explorations. Therapeutic change also rests on this notion. The way we have been doing it (in some cases over and over for decades) no longer works well, so we seek help to change what we have been doing. For this, we need novel experiences, but not just any novel experiences—ones that emerge from bodyful states.

We often fear novelty because it almost always involves a gap. We must let go of an old identity or an old way of doing something and step into the unknown. This is likely why organized religions tend to invoke faith. Having faith, particularly a faith shared with others, helps with this gap and helps us step into the unknown without too much fear or dissociation, and sometimes even with a sense of curiosity and wonder.

How does our body find and keep faith? It does so by staying awake and engaged in the gaps. This goes back to our understanding of attention and of goal-oriented and non-goal-oriented movement. Faith's bodyful ingredients are our oscillations of attention and our oscillations between goal-oriented and non-goal-oriented actions. In the midst of the rapids of change, our attention sharpens, and it moves between our body—how it's positioned in space—and the nature of the space around us. This is exactly what my canoe instructor did in the white water—he felt his body and its relationship to the canoe, and he observed the water, the rocks, and the banks of the river. By oscillating his attention between them, he associated them to each other. By experiencing these elements as an interactive system, he was able to be an engaged part of that system. He played with small, rapid responses—an angling of the paddle, a slight lean to the left. He found effective actions and quickly abandoned ones that didn't work. In the midst of navigating change, we oscillate between goal-oriented experiments and letting go of goals when they start to "push the river."

In the next section, after working with pressure, pleasure, and inquiry exercises, we will work with a very serious, advanced change practice called the Goofy practice. Goofy, as you may know, is a cartoon dog invented by Walt Disney. He's big, completely clumsy, relentlessly cheerful, and always sticking his nose into current events. He's not a big thinker or planner. Exuberantly inept, playfully experimental, and completely devoid of self-consciousness, he lives for novel experiences. We will use several of his characteristics as inspiration for our novelty practice. It's important not to get too stuffy about building this skill, as that will monotonize the practice.

Practices for Pressure

- *Listening to symptoms.* Clear some time and space, and begin with oscillating your attention, inside and outside, for a minute or two to wake up your attentional muscles. Now turn your attention to inner body sensations, and find a sensation that you might describe as a small pain or uncomfortable place. Don't choose intense pains unless you feel you can work with the intensity of what might arise. If you don't notice any symptoms of small pain, put yourself in an awkward or unusual position. This usually wakes up a tight muscle you can then work with. Begin by focusing on the "symptom" sensation, just observing it but not judging or trying to explain it. Notice the subtle details of the sensation and what it does when you breathe or move slightly. Don't try to relieve the sensation; rather, listen to it just as it is. Work to accept its presence by turning toward it with your attention and care. You can stay with this practice as a kind of meditation or you can go on to the next exercise.

- *Giving symptoms a voice.* After listening to the sensation without judgment or analysis, begin to imagine that this sensation is a kind of nonverbal statement your body is making. You may want to find a sound that expresses it as accurately as possible. Notice what associations come up with the sensation or the sound: images, colors, other sensations, emotions, memories. Hold these associations in your attention along with the original sensation. See if a word emerges that expresses the sensation and your associations, and say that word out loud. If it feels right, see if this sensation can put a few words together that express how it feels right now. If any of these words sound analytical, judgmental, explanatory, or dismissive, identify this as "finding the wrong voice" and go back to just observing the sensation and associations. We want the pain to talk rather than have our cognitive self talk to the pain or about the pain. When the pain begins to talk on its own terms, we often access feelings, upsets, and memories that we haven't acknowledged before. You can stop here by acknowledging the voice or go on to the next practice.

- *Moving the voice.* Now ask the sensation, the associations, and the voice a question: "How do you want to move with this feeling?" Give the experience a gesture along with any sounds and words. Trust how the sensation wants to move you; perhaps it wants to curl you over, clench your jaw, or get you up to jump around. Allow the sensation to roll over into an action, done deliberately, with breath and ongoing sensory tracking. Often by letting these movements sequence—go where they want to go—the pain can communicate itself, and its experience can be felt as well as understood. Often these movements represent parts of ourselves that we haven't been communicating with. Our ability to let this part of ourselves be visible and be somatically honest can open the door to resolutions we didn't "think" possible. You can rest here, or stop, or go on to the next practice.

- *Experimenting with novel meaning.* The meaning we derive from an experience comes after fully engaging with it; otherwise we are just making up explanations that may or may not have much to do with what is really going on. This is why in bodyfulness practices we work to postpone meaning making until after a movement sequence is complete. We want unexplored, novel parts of us to contribute to the new narrative that might emerge from the experience. So after the movement sequencing above feels finished for now (it may need multiple movings in order to feel completely finished), take a few minutes to rest back into attending to sensation, noticing any ways your body might now feel different. Let your focus get a bit dreamy; don't try hard to find meaning—let your sense of what this experience means to you emerge slowly and inclusively. Whatever ideas begin to emerge about experience, see them as neither true nor false but as a narrative that you can work with for as long as it feels useful. You may want to write it down. The stories that coalesce from our bodyful experiences are maps of our inner terrain and its relationship to outer locations. As such, they are not the territories themselves but guides as we travel through our lives.

- *Touch and go.* In Buddhist psychology, therapists use a practice called *touch and go*, where they guide the client to work with a painful state by touching it with their attention and care and then resting away from the hard work of engaging with the pain. In this way the client oscillates their efforts and avoids getting overwhelmed. Next time you are experiencing some pain, try this back-and-forth engagement. The task is to gently touch a sore feeling with care and compassion and then put your attention elsewhere. This creates a metabenefit of exercising the muscle of attention so that it gets stronger and more capable.

Practices for Pleasure

- *Finding natural pleasures.* Clear some time and space to experiment with this practice, trusting that you will know how long
you want to spend with it. Only do this practice for as long as
you can tolerate and enjoy these natural pleasures. Start by
oscillating your attention in and out for a bit. Then begin to
focus in and out on pleasant things—the way the light comes
through a window or the pleasant feeling of a full stomach.
Purposefully land your attention on parts of your body that
feel well and on elements of the room that please you. Notice
how this is working. Is it difficult? Easy? Does it change your
mood in some way? Now let's add in movement. Take a few
minutes to do self-touch in ways that feel positive and pleasant. It could be a gentle stroke on your lower arm, a scalp
scratch, or a rub of your calf—whatever feels good. Make sure
to put your attention to the feeling response so that the pleasant touch becomes active and you really absorb the pleasant
sensations. Notice what associations arise. Is there any way
you are limiting your enjoyment of this simple, natural pleasure? Experiment with this practice, finding different body locations, such as the back of your knee or your earlobe. You can
stop here or move on to the next practice.

- *Learning to play.* Find a position that feels comfortable: standing, sitting, or lying down. Take the next bit of time to make a
commitment to move, and to only move in ways that feel pleasant or fun. You may be surprised at how challenging this can
be. It harkens back to the physical play of children, when they
spontaneously erupt in jumps, waves, and wiggles. As adults,

we can do that, but we have more options. It can be a slow, luxurious stretch of your arms that feels just right. It can be dancing to music. It can involve moves that just feel playful to you—making funny faces, getting into a contorted position, or making odd noises. Take some minutes to spontaneously and physically play while you keep your attention on your body— what it feels, where it is, and what it wants to do next. What associations come up? When you feel finished, take a minute or two to track your inner sensations and note how you feel physically and emotionally.

- *Learning to play with others.* This exercise requires one play-mate who is willing to physically play with you, but it can be adapted for more than two players. Clear a space where all of you can move around easily and safely. A few ground rules: During the practice, don't converse in ways that take you out of the physical play practice. It would be best to avoid talking altogether. No touching in ways that feel unwelcome to the person being touched. Respect your partners' limits about how the playing unfolds (some people, for instance, love to wrestle while others don't). Begin by facing each other. One person makes a spontaneous movement, such as a funny face, a wave, or a shoulder shrug. The partner responds—it doesn't have to be the same movement—and then you respond in whatever way your body impulse impels you. You can stay with this trading of motions back and forth, or you can just let it go where it wants to go—around the room, into dancing together or playful pushing. The idea is to have fun, to learn to read each other's play signals, to get a feeling for your limits of what is fun, as well as theirs, and find things to do that please you both.

Afterward, talk about it together. Relational play can bring up buried assumptions about how relationships work, about power, and about when fun feels threatening. Just listen to one another and appreciate each other for the play practice.

Practices for Inquiry

- *Reducing goal-oriented movements.* We might consider these next practices advanced because we tend to be unfamiliar with finding and working with seemingly purposeless motion. We get a good start in spontaneous play, but now we want to apply a similar creative impulsiveness to our inquiry practice, where we let go of where a movement usually goes next and turn away from goals to work with certain states, such as pain and pleasure. We can begin with a simple exercise we have done before. Sitting comfortably, put your attention into your left or right lower arm and hand. Take a minute to oscillate your attention between looking at your lower arm and sensing it from the inside. Now let it begin to move in any way it wants. The arm could rotate, as could the wrist. The hand can flex or twist. The trick here is to slow it down and move in ways that you can't predict. For instance, if you curl your hand into a fist, would you then predict that you will stretch and extend it? Keep oscillating your attention between looking at your hand and feeling it, and playing with not being as predictable in your actions. You can stop here or go on to the next practice.

- *Focusing on non-goal-oriented movements (movement inquiry practice).* We noted earlier that Sigmund Freud pioneered the idea of free association, during which we engage in a kind of off-the-cuff speaking that wanders without needing to make sense, so as to access unconscious thoughts and feelings. We are going to work at greater depth now with physical free association. Clear a time and space where you can move around, and begin, in any position, by doing any physical self-care you like, or you can start by practicing the pressure or pleasure work. After a few minutes, let your body get quiet, and rest your attention on the details of the sensations your body is experiencing. Wait as long as it takes for an impulse to move in some way. It might be a micromovement or it might move around the room. The idea is to let go and be moved rather than willing yourself to move. It may feel that no impulses to move arise, or that it's hard to distinguish between goal-oriented and non-goal-oriented motions. No worries. Practice will help you sort these things out. Just keep your attention on your body and imagine movement that has no reason, just itself, moving.

The Goofy Practice

- *Letting yourself be odd and spontaneous.* The Goofy practice often feels playful and fun, such that it often helps us with increasing our tolerance for natural pleasures. Goofy has a natural affinity for play, but this practice can also be applied to the pressure and inquiry domains as well. Trust what shows up. Trust how your body channels Goofy. Find a space and time where you can move around freely. One of the best ways to begin is to get into a strange position that feels odd—whatever your body is able to do. You wouldn't want to do this position in public. It can be as simple as bending over and looking behind you through your legs or as complex as twisting yourself into a human pretzel. You can also experiment with strange sounds or odd looks on your face. Assume that this position is a very advanced meditation position and just stay awake to it, noticing the details of your experience and enjoying the novelty. You can extend the practice by taking it into motion, playing with getting around in the room in that position. Notice the associations and thoughts that arise. Acknowledge them, and then return to the practice.

- *Goofing around together.* This practice, done with other goofy people, echoes the exercise above, with the addition of staying in relationship to another or others while doing it. Notice the relational dynamics that show up, and notice when your attention goes away from the practice. Acknowledge that and move on.

10

The Enlightened Body

ENLIGHTENMENT CAN BE a tricky term. It typically denotes someone who is fully awake all the time—fully aware and attentive—a state that is said to bring suffering to an end. In Eastern wisdom traditions, one can achieve full awakeness and sustain it all the time while still in this body, though only a few have been said to have achieved this state. However, most wisdom teachers in the East explain that we enter and exit moments of enlightenment and that our task while "in this body" is to make efforts to increase our percentage of awakened moments and to work for this state in others. Yet trying hard to be fully enlightened can work against itself, as trying can take you out of the present moment, away from engagement with it.

So what do we work for while we are here? Regardless of whether we believe that some noncorporeal part of ourselves survives death, our embodied life task seems to include conscious efforts to reduce suffering, both in ourselves and in the world, as well as to promote our happiness and the happiness of others. We have looked at bodyfulness as a means to accomplish this task and seen the literal and metaphoric ways in which personal and sociocultural bodies move in and out of awakened states. We have also seen that there will always be parts of ourselves outside of our awareness, areas of our body that move with the pulsations of life in ways that we can co-operate with and feel grateful for. We have worked with practices that can guide us in challenging and extending our body's experiences in disciplined and playful ways. As a result of these ideas and practices, we can increase our percentage of bodyful moments, and this carries the possibility of "lightening up." We can be happier. Our body can be happier, quite literally, and it can act in ways that assist other bodies in being happier.

In an old *Star Trek: The Next Generation* episode, Captain Picard encounters a race of aliens that address the crew as "ugly bags of mostly water." This is their definition of human, their wry view of human bodies. While technically true that we contain mostly water, the human body does amazing things with that water. As a way of reviewing our understanding of bodyfulness, let's look at what our watery body does that we can make use of in order to be more awake and happier, as whatever body we are—given to us by our ancestors, nurtured by our caregivers, and moving through life right now under our own power.

- *We oscillate.* We move along multiple body continuums—from minimal to expansive—constantly. Bodyfulness asks us to wake up to and engage with these physical, emotional, cognitive, and attentional continuums more purposefully. By doing so, we navigate into and out of awakened states with increasing alacrity and grace. When we oscillate along continuums, we have less interest in creating categories that separate things and critiquing the differences. When we oscillate more consciously and deliberately, we expand our behavioral repertoire—from physical to emotional to social—and we athleticize our mobility, our ability to move in any needed direction.

- *We balance.* We poise ourselves over and around certain set points and places, from metabolic to sociocultural identities. This balancing practice might be how the body works with stillness, that while relatively quiet nonetheless involves constantly adjusting micromovements. The athleticism of this practice helps us find our stability and our current location (here and now), a reference point crucial to our sense of being. Together, oscillation and balance pair up to create semipermeable boundaries and a fluid sense of self.

- *We inter-are.* We began with the interior of our body and saw that all of what lies inside us works as a network, an interconnected and interdependent grouping that gets things done because it works as a symphony does, creating our complex and rich body song. So too, we are connected to and interdependent with other organisms and, by extension, all existence. Understanding this truth helps us more consciously cooperate with all our feedback loops, from local sensorimotor and viscerolimbic feedback loops to distant systems far outside our personal body. By acknowledging and engaging with this reality, we form a more gut-level sense of connection to ourselves and others, a more activated orientation to other's well-being, and a means of relating bodyfully to all.

- *We repeat things and we change things.* Things that bear repeating— actions that serve the health and well-being of any organism—

are programmed into the body as automatic actions that operate below conscious awareness as cellular and metabolic oscillations. For this we can feel grateful to our ancestors and for the deep time that evolution has had to perfect this energy-conserving aliveness. In our embodied middle ground, we have limited influence over semiautomatic actions and events, such as breathing and heart rate, as well as actions by others around us. On the other end of the continuum we experiment, we change things up, and we play spontaneously with what life sends our way. From acknowledging that which we currently have no control over, and working bodyfully with this truth, all the way to creating something from scratch, we can relax into our varying levels of control over what happens. By consciously and purposefully finding our location along this continuum, we can deal with change as it washes over us. We can also appreciate the grace of actions that know what to do without our conscious engagement, as these represent our basic and communal aliveness. And we can challenge ourselves to change the things we can by using bodyfulness as a friendly influence.

- *We associate.* Bodyfulness begins when we find associations, more than explanations, for our experiences and others' actions. Explanations tend to box up events in ways that more or less distort the power and meaning of lived experience. Associations arise from the bottom-up sensations and feelings of our body. Associations help us uncover buried meanings that may no longer serve us, as well as show us how we really feel about something. They push back against overthinking. Only by listening to these body-based signals can we "make sense" of our experiences in ways that then blend with thought to construct usable models of ourselves and the world. In this way we generate both physical and behavioral integrity. When we work from the wisdom of felt experience as it then blends with thoughtful reflection, we generate an experience of wholeness, similar to the wholeness we refer to when we talk about preserving the integrity of our body and others' bodies.

- *We breathe, move, sense, and relate.* Bodyfulness rests on these four practice pillars, the ongoing actions that require our attention and purpose in order to live a bodyful life. When we breathe consciously as an ongoing practice, we gradually influence ingrained mechanisms that manage our energy levels, metabolism, and emotions. When we move our body on purpose—as a means of synchronizing ourselves with our inner micromovements, revealing an emotion, or playing exuberantly—we athleticize our ability to feel more empowered in our life, to communicate meaningfully with others, to be creative, and to be a graceful activist. In particular, movement allows us to experiment along the continuum from habit to novelty and challenge ourselves at various points along this expanse as a way to increase our ability to make good use of each. When we sense ourselves as we move, attending carefully to the nuanced voices inside us, outside us, and at our borders, we gather some of our most useful and pragmatic information about *what is*, and we athleticize our attentional muscles in ways that keep our sensory filters freer of the flotsam of unconscious bias. Thus, with a more focused lens on the present moment, breathing, sensing, and moving allow us to relate to others contactfully. They enable us to lovingly dance closer to and farther away from others in ways that allow us to celebrate our mutual, semipermeable selves.

- *We play.* Play constitutes one of our earliest and most enduring methods for bodyful practice because of its ties to neuroplasticity, healing, sociality, physicality, and natural, active pleasure. Play challenges the status quo and allows us to leverage change through positive states. Importantly, play needs to emerge from our breathing, moving, sensing, and relating, where it can be crafted from what our body is naturally inclined to do that feels fun. It illustrates the profound healing power of the creative act, whether that act be a cartwheel, a ball tossed to a teammate, or an improvisation on a guitar.

- *We narrate our stories.* Finding and expressing our body stories, alongside attending to the body narratives of others, allow us to bear witness to the sorrows and joys of human and nonhuman existence. Completing the whole sequence of a body story helps us feel more at peace with it and positions it as a meaningful remembrance rather than a repetitive compulsion. When we attend to body stories of trauma, oppression, and neglect, whether in ourselves or others, we foster a type of activism that enables us to use our moving body as a force for recovery and reparation. We realize our connection to others—whether in sorrow, anger, joy, or delight—when we move together in mutually constructed body narratives. Bodyfulness tells, retells, and renegotiates our body memories in ways that cause us to be more wakeful and reflective. In this way we directly experience and appreciate our multiple, mutable identities via our ongoing narratives.

- *We practice.* Bodyfulness can be seen as inherently accessible and cultivated through disciplined practice. Just like in the body itself, contemplative fitness occurs via both freestanding and embedded actions that attend to, engage with, acknowledge, and integrate the body's experiences. The idea of fitness as a harbinger of bodyfulness can be interpreted via our own bodily authority, such that it involves not only sweaty exercise but also a gentle caress and attentiveness to a painful or pleasurable sensation. As far as the body is concerned, patterns of use structure many of our subsequent experiences. This holds true for the heart and brain as well as muscles. The good news is that bodyful practice can undo, redo, and reinforce bodily experiences through directed and nondirected means. And there is no prepackaged system of practice that we have to buy into in order to achieve bodyfulness. Many wonderful practices from many different traditions already exist that can be used to wake up our body. Other practices we can wisely adapt, and still others we can make up on our own.

We have experimented with inventing a new word that, by its use, centralizes an undervalued and underdeveloped essence of who we are right now, right here. We have seen that human capacities long associated with mindfulness, such as attention, awareness, and present-centeredness, are actually rooted in the flesh and can't occur without the body's actions. While sitting on a cushion or kneeling in prayer brings with it many health benefits and contemplative insights, how we get up off the cushion, floor, or pew and navigate our daily life requires the breathing, moving, sensing, and relating body. Reflection without action doesn't change anything because the feedback loop of contemplative inner experience and contemplative outer action demands that we stay the course, that we stay with the sequence such that our body literally enacts its awakened state. Only then is enlightenment truly a light in the world, one that shines both inward and outward.

How will you find and practice your bodyfulness? Because of its bottom-up roots, the practice of bodyfulness develops from the authority of your lived experience rather than being handed down to you, prepackaged, from a master. Your body knows how to wake up. You only have to attend to its signals, actively include the associations that emerge, move with body memories that need to complete, and allow present-moment movement inquiries to inform you as to your direction. From here, you step out into your daily life with not only ideas but also bodily capabilities. While this can be a daunting task, the results can be stunning. And when challenges result in a sense of satisfaction, completion, and accomplishment, our happiness home-grows as a result of our efforts.

We can always study and share faith with masterful people, in ways that give us experiential input we can then form into our own practices. But by trusting our bodily integrity and authority, we become much more capable of resisting oppression, autocracy, and abuses of power from wherever they may originate. In current geopolitical circumstances, this skill may be increasingly needed. Bodyfulness sits squarely in our outer world as well as our inner experience. This outer world, for most of us, tends to valorize how the body appears rather than how it's experienced. It tends to commodify our body, domesticate it, ignore it, and shame it. Bodyfulness pushes back against these forces. Bodyfulness breeds an active life, and this activism can take many creative and contributive forms. You know best.

At its heart, bodyfulness is a contemplative practice. Yet contemplation and action inter-are, as we have seen so many times. Practice can and should occur in specialized, often sacred circumstances, yet bodyfulness, while making use of many freestanding practices, finds its home in our embedded experiences of daily living. *Embedded practice* may be another good synonym for bodyfulness. How we reach out to pick up our child, how we wait before eating to check to see if we are really hungry, how we gaze at a troubled stranger, how we notice a gut feeling, and how we breathe into a happy moment—all these experiences can be bodyful. We access this bodyful state by practicing right now, during this breath, feeling this sensation, noticing this small motion. Right here. Right now.

Chapter Practices

- Go back through the book, choose one of your favorite practices, and do it again, noticing if any changes have occurred. What makes this practice a favorite? Then choose one that was fairly challenging or seemingly odd, and do it again. Notice what associations arise and hold them in your attention without judgment or analysis. What made this practice challenging?

- Take one of the practices in this book and adapt it as an experiment. See how your changes take it in a different direction and what that different direction feels like.

- Remember a physical exercise or practice that you have learned from others that has been useful to you. It could be a stretch, pose, movement sequence, or sensory practice. Notice what it is like to do it in ways you consider bodyful.

- Using your body authority, feel free to make up a bodyfulness practice of your own and notice where it takes you physically, emotionally, and mentally. You may want to write it down and over time perfect it with small or large tweaks. Enjoy!

Appendix A

The Body's Organs and Their Functions

Organs are structures that each have a definite shape and function and are composed of two or more types of tissues.

ORGAN	ORGAN FUNCTION	ORGAN LOCATION
Brain	Control center of the nervous system	Inside the skull
Lungs	Provide oxygen to bloodstream and exhale carbon dioxide	Inside the chest cavity
Liver	Processes contents of blood—break down fats, produce urea, filter harmful substances, maintain glucose levels	Right side of abdominal cavity, beneath diaphragm
Bladder	Stores and releases urine	Pelvic cavity
Kidneys	Maintain body's chemical balance by excreting waste and excess fluid	Back of abdominal cavity, one on each side of spinal column
Heart	Pumps blood through blood vessels	Chest cavity

Stomach	Digests food through production of gastric juices that break down food into a thin liquid	Lying crosswise in abdominal cavity, beneath diaphragm
Intestines	Small intestine: absorbs most digested food Large intestine: absorbs water and excretes solid waste	Between stomach and anus—divided into small and large portions

Appendix B

The Body's Systems and Their Functions

A system is comprised of an association of organs that have a common function.

SYSTEM	STRUCTURES INVOLVED	SYSTEM FUNCTION
Circulatory	Heart, blood, blood vessels, arteries, veins	Moves blood, nutrients, oxygen, carbon dioxide, and hormones throughout body
Digestive	Mouth, esophagus, stomach, gallbladder, small intestine, large intestine, rectum, and anus	Breaks down and absorbs food and removes waste
Endocrine	Pituitary, thyroid, parathyroid, thymus, adrenals, pancreas, ovaries, testicles	Secretes hormones into blood, which regulates body functions (metabolism, growth, sexual)
Immune	Lymph nodes, spleen, bone marrow, lymphocytes (B and T cells), and leukocytes (white blood cells)	Defends against bacteria, viruses, and other pathogens

Lymphatic	Lymph nodes, lymph ducts, lymph vessels	Makes and moves lymph, removes excess lymph and returns it to blood
Nervous	Central: brain, spinal cord Peripheral: nerves	Controls voluntary and involuntary action, sends and receives signals from every part of body
Muscular	Muscles (skeletal, smooth, cardiac)	Aids movement, supports posture, blood flow
Reproductive	Vagina, uterus, ovaries, penis, testes	Allows reproduction (produces and delivers gametes, nourishes young)
Skeletal	Bones, tendons, ligaments, cartilage, teeth	Supports movement, stores calcium and blood cells, protects organs, maintains posture
Integumentary	Skin, hair, nails	Protects from outside world, regulates temperature, eliminates waste (perspiration), synthesizes vitamin D, senses touch, prevents dehydration
Urinary	Kidneys, ureters, bladder, sphincter muscles, urethra	Eliminates waste (urea), helps regulate blood pressure and volume and electrolyte balance, regulates acid-base homeostasis
Respiratory	Trachea, diaphragm, lungs	Takes in oxygen, expels carbon dioxide, creates sound through air vibration, supports smelling

Appendix C
The Types of Sensations

Sensation can be technically defined as the electrochemical excitation of a sensory nerve and the registration of this incoming impulse by the brain. The processing and categorizing of this sensation by the brain is often called *perception*.

There are several different ways to classify sensations. Typically sensory neurons are classified by their physical form, where they are located in the body, and the specialized functions they perform. One way to classify them is by what type of stimuli they respond to. A few examples:

- *Chemoreceptors* detect the presence of chemicals.

- *Thermoreceptors* detect changes of temperature.

- *Mechanoreceptors* detect mechanical forces (movement, tension, pressure).

- *Photoreceptors* detect light.

- *Nociceptors* detect damage or threat to tissues and create pain responses.

- *Baroreceptors* detect levels of pressure in blood vessels.

Different animals have different types of sensory neurons, though many types are shared by most species. For instance, some animals have receptors that can pick up infrared light; humans don't have those, so we can't pick up that type of stimuli. Different species have differing amounts of certain receptors—dogs' sense of smell is better than ours, eagles have acuter vision. The takeaway idea here is that the world is a lot bigger than what we sense it to be.

Given all the different types of sensory neurons, it helps to clump them together according to general principles. The list below represents our current efforts to categorize sensation:

- *Proprioception.* These are our sensations of movement, body position, balance, and orientation in space. The term *kinesthesia* has been used interchangeably with *proprioception*, though the term *kinesthesia* tends to place more emphasis on body motion and less emphasis on balance. The sensory neurons for proprioception sit inside the inner ear as well as in and around various joints in the body. These sensations give us a reading of our location in relationship to the outer world and from one part of the body to another. These senses get stimulated when we roll around, hang upside down, somersault, and, in general, play. The ability to use proprioceptors well has been correlated to the ability to focus and sustain attention.

- *Exteroception.* These are sensors in our nose, eyes, ears, and skin that pick up stimuli from the outside world. They tend to be located near or on the surface of the body. People with sensory processing disorders (such as autism) tend to have problems with how these neurons work, such that they tend to experience "typical" levels of sound, light, and touch as overwhelming. Some people believe that modern technological living has overemphasized these senses, unbalancing us in fundamental ways.

- *Interoception.* These are the senses that gather data about our internal world, the inside of our body. Examples would be hunger, thirst, sexual arousal, and feeling hot or cold, as well as more general feelings such as queasiness, sleepiness, breathing, and heart rate. The ability to track inner sensation has been correlated to the ability to track and understand our emotions and thus our emotional intelligence.

We often equate interoception with *body awareness*, though proprioception and even exteroception should be included in our understanding of body awareness as well. Our literal sense of self arises from a combination of these three types of sensing, as well as our movements or actions (our sensorimotor loop). This is why this book emphasizes practices that balance different types of sensation in concert with different types of action as vital components of a bodyful life.

Notes

Introduction

1. Genji Sugamura, at Kansai University in Japan, has used the term at two different conferences in 2006 and 2007, around the same time I began informally using it in my classroom.

2. Yuasa Yasuo, *The Body: Toward an Eastern Mind-Body Theory* (New York: SUNY Press, 1987).

3. Materialism in the eighteenth and nineteenth centuries was strongly influenced by the mechanization that occurred during the Industrial Revolution, as well as the teachings of Darwin, who pointed out that we are a type of animal, that is, not separate from other life-forms.

4. Marika Tiggemann, "Media Influences on Body Image Development," in *Body Image: A Handbook of Theory, Research, and Clinical Practice*, eds. Thomas F. Cash and Thomas Pruzinsky (New York: Guilford Press, 2002).

Chapter 2: The Anatomy of Bodyfulness

1. See Martha Eddy, *Mindful Movement: The Evolution of the Somatic Arts and Conscious Action* (Chicago: Intellect Press, 2016).

Chapter 3: Sensing

1. Kinesthesia is sometimes equated with the term *proprioception*. The term *proprioception* sometimes is made distinct from kinesthesia by adding in our sense of balance.

2. We have several types of muscles in the body. For instance, the heart is a muscle, but it's not attached to a bone. There is also muscular action going on in the gut. These are called smooth muscles.

3. A. Jean Ayres, *Sensory Integration and Learning Disorders* (Los Angeles, CA: Western Psychological Services, 1973).

Chapter 4: Breathing

1. Shortly after achieving earth orbit, an accidental explosion disabled the machine that removed the carbon dioxide from the astronauts' air supply. Their exhales, rich in CO_2, soon created a life-threatening imbalance of gases, which they heroically solved by making a new CO_2 scrubber out of found objects in the capsule.

2. I first published a version of this practice in coauthorship with Victoria Himmat Kaur, "Breathwork in Body Psychotherapy: Clinical Applications," *Body, Movement, and Dance in Psychotherapy* 8, no. 4 (April 2013): 216–28, https://doi.org/10.1080/17432979.2013.828657.

3. I learned this image of the ribs resting closer to each other from Judith Aston, developer of Aston-Patterning, a movement education and bodywork form. See www.astonkinetics.com.

Chapter 5: Moving

1. Body-Mind Centering, a movement education system, pays a lot of attention to these fundamental actions, as well as to reflexes. If you want to pursue this avenue, I would recommend this system. See www.bodymindcentering.com.

2. Structural and functional holding are terms popularized by Judith Aston, developer of Aston-Patterning. See www.astonkinetics.com.

Chapter 6: Relating

1. This research can be found in Tiffany Field, *Touch* (Cambridge, MA: MIT Press, 2003).

2. One of my favorite definitions of a parent is put forth by Allan N. Schore, in his seminal book *Affect Regulation and the Origins of the Self* (Mahwah, NJ: Lawrence Erlbaum Associates, 1994). He calls parents "external psychobiological regulators." The parent externally regulates the child until they can manage it themselves, physically, emotionally, and mentally.

3. Mark L. Knapp and Judith A. Hall, *Nonverbal Communication in Human Interaction* (Belmont, CA: Thomson Higher Education, 2006).

4. This positive regulation stands in contrast to evidence that we can also form negative attunements and attachments to people, sometimes called trauma bonding, where we influence each other to become less regulated, less healthy. For this reason we need the skill of breaking off attunement as well as engaging in it.

5. If you have never done sitting meditation, it may be best to simply work toward quieting your mind, where you observe your direct experience. Every time you notice yourself thinking, just label that a "thought" and go back to wordlessly observing your direct experience.

Chapter 7: Body Identity, Body Authority, and Bodyful Stories

1. Hubert J. M. Hermans, "The Dialogical Self: Toward a Theory of Personal and Cultural Positioning," *Culture and Psychology* 7, no. 3 (2001): 248.

2. This practice owes a lot of its inspiration to a dance therapy form called Authentic Movement. See authenticmovementcommunity.org.

Chapter 8: Bodylessness and the Reclamation of Bodily Authority

1. Frank Newport, "In U.S., 42% Believe Creationist View of Human Origins," *Gallup*, news.gallup.com/poll/170822/believe-credentialist-view-human-origins.aspx.

2. Max Weisbuch and Kristin Pauker, "The Nonverbal Transmission of Intergroup Bias: A Model of Bias Contagion with Implications for Social Policy," *Social Issues and Policy Review* 5, no. 1 (December 2011): 257–91.

3. Both of these writers can be found in *Oppression and the Body: Roots, Resistance, and Resolution*, edited by Christine Caldwell and Bennett Leighton (Berkeley, CA: North Atlantic Books, 2018).

4. You might want to check out the Implicit Assumption Test (IAT), developed to test for unconscious forms of bias. The test is online, confidential, and doesn't take long. Enter this term into a search engine and you will find it. Notice that several of the tests have to do with our unconscious assumptions about bodies.

5. Martin Luther King Jr., "Where Do We Go From Here?" (sermon, 11th Annual Southern Christian Leadership Conference, Atlanta, GA, August 16, 1967).

6. Ibid.

7. Ibid. In the same sermon, Martin Luther King Jr. noted that love without power is sentimental and anemic, and that power without love is reckless and abusive.

Chapter 9: When Being Here Takes You There

1. Four prominent therapies fit this description: dialectical behavioral therapy, mindfulness-based stress reduction, mindfulness-based cognitive therapy, and acceptance and commitment therapy.

2. Research has shown that exercise and social support are just as effective as antidepressants for most mild to moderate depressions, with beneficial rather than harmful side effects.

3. *Flow* is a term popularized by Mihaly Csikszentmihalyi, a professor and researcher at the University of Chicago.

Additional Notes
and References

THIS SECTION INCLUDES publishing information for sources mentioned in the book, cites additional resources and references, and briefly explains more technical details of some of the covered concepts. It's organized according to chapter and topics within those chapters.

Introduction

Mindfulness increasing immune function and lessening stress. Ruth A. Baer, James Carmody, and Matthew Hunsinger, "Weekly Change in Mindfulness and Perceived Stress in a Mindfulness-Based Stress Reduction Program," *Journal of Clinical Psychology* 68, no. 7 (July 2012): 755–65, doi:10.1002/jclp.21865.

Mindfulness lessening disorders of attention. Jan M. Burg, Oliver T. Wolf, and Johannes Michalak, "Mindfulness as Self-Regulated Attention: Associations with Heart Rate Variability," *Swiss Journal of Psychology* 71, no. 3 (January 2012): 135–39.

Mindfulness lessening mental and emotional illness. Philippe R. Goldin and James J. Gross, "Effects of Mindfulness-Based Stress Reduction (MBSR) on Emotion Regulation in Social Anxiety Disorder," *Emotion* 10, no. 1 (February 2010): 83–91; also, Sheryl M. Green and Peter J. Bieling, "Expanding the Scope of Mindfulness-Based Cognitive Therapy: Evidence for Effectiveness in a Heterogeneous Psychiatric Sample," *Cognitive and Behavioral Practice* 19, no. 1 (2012): 174–80, doi:10.1016/j.cbpra.2011.02.006.

Heightened somatic awareness. Thomas Hanna, *Somatics: Reawakening the Mind's Control of Movement, Flexibility, and Health* (New York: Addison-Wesley Company, 1988); Thomas Hanna, *The Body of Life* (New York: Alfred A. Knopf, 1979); Don Hanlon Johnson, *Body, Spirit and Democracy* (Berkeley: North Atlantic Books, 1994).

Body sense. Alan Fogel, *The Psychophysiology of Self-Awareness: Rediscovering the Lost Art of Body Sense* (New York: W.W. Norton, 2009).

Somaesthetics. Richard Shusterman, *Body Consciousness: A Philosophy of Mindfulness and Somaesthetics* (New York: Cambridge University Press, 2008).

Embodied and enactive cognition. Shaun Gallagher, "Phenomenology and Embodied Cognition," in *The Routledge Handbook of Embodied Cognition*, ed. Lawrence Shapiro (London: Routledge, 2014), 9–18.

Wordlessly shared intersubjective relating and knowing. Diana Fosha, *The Transforming Power of Affect: A Model for Accelerated Change* (New York: Basic Books, 2002); Daniel N. Stern, *The Present Moment in Psychotherapy and Everyday Life* (New York: W.W. Norton, 2004).

Body to body transmission of healing. Margaret Wilkinson, *Changing Minds in Therapy: Emotion, Attachment, Trauma, and Neurobiology* (New York: W.W. Norton, 2010).

Negative emotional response to one's silhouette. Linda Jackson, "Physical Attractiveness: A Sociocultural Perspective," in *Body Image: A Handbook of Theory, Research, and Clinical Practice*, ed. Thomas F. Cash and Thomas Pruzinsky (New York: Guilford Press, 2002), 13–21.

Materialism. John Kaag, *American Philosophy: A Love Story* (New York: Farrar, Straus and Giroux, 2016).

Mindfulness-based stress reduction (MBSR). Beginning in the mid-1980s, researchers and clinicians such as Jon Kabat-Zinn et al. (1985), using clinical trials, have found that mindfulness meditation reduced physical pain, negative body image, mood disturbances, anxiety, and depression, as well as increased self-esteem. Kabat-Zinn and others speculated that because the practice was inexpensive to teach, because it stressed self-observation and self-responsibility, and because participants used it under their own control, that it also enhanced insight and self-worth. Numerous other studies have found that MBSR positively effects both cognitive and affective processing (Ramel et al., 2004).

Body-mind research. When research looking at mind-body medicine or mind-body therapies is reviewed, findings tend to replicate the lessening of pain, decreased anxiety and depression, and improvements in ADHD symptoms seen in meditation research.

Chapter 1: The Eight Core Principles of Bodyfulness

Physics, mass, energy, and oscillations. Trying to grasp basic physics can be daunting, but luckily there are many great popular books on the matter (and on matter) and some great YouTube videos. On YouTube, I would recommend any public lecture by any of the following: Brian Greene, Neil Turok, Lawrence Krauss, Sean Carroll, Michio Kaku, Brian Cox, and Frank Wilczek. These are folks who specialize in making physics and cosmology accessible to the public in very interesting ways. In terms of books, if you want to really dig into the science I would recommend: Carlo Rovelli, *Seven Brief Lessons on Physics* (New York: Riverhead Books, 2016); Steven Weinberg, *To Explain the World: The Discovery of Modern Science* (New York: Harper Perennial, 2016).

The mind in every cell of the body, and emotion as cellular regulation. Candace B. Pert, *Molecules of Emotion: The Science Behind Mind-Body Medicine* (New York: Touchstone, 1999).

Attention or concentration. A classic text: B. Alan Wallace, *The Attention Revolution: Unlocking the Power of the Focused Mind* (Boston: Wisdom Publications,

2006). Another classic text: Arthur J. Deikman, *The Observing Self: Mysticism and Psychotherapy* (Boston: Beacon Press, 1983).

Presentness. Daniel N. Stern, *The Present Moment in Psychotherapy and Everyday Life* (New York: W.W. Norton, 2004). Another excellent text, especially if you like reading about the brain: Daniel J. Siegel, *The Mindful Brain: Reflection and Attunement in the Cultivation of Well-Being* (New York: W.W. Norton Publishers, 2007).

Neuroplasticity. If you want to investigate neuroplasticity, I recommend Norman Doidge, *The Brain That Changes Itself* (New York: Penguin, 2007). It's an easy and interesting read.

Movement awareness and education. There are many good movement education systems that work with energy conservation and the process of changing problematic body habits via contrasting experiences. One is the Feldenkrais Method, a body education system that teaches you to select useful movement and inhibit "parasitic" muscle contractions that can cause fatigue and stress. You have to sense the old action first in order to then inhibit or select it. A useful website is https://ISMETA.org if you want to get a sense of some of the different movement education systems.

Unconscious emotional processing. Regarding our already feeling an emotion before we are aware of it: This was first discovered by a researcher named Benjamin Libet (1999), who found that people become aware of an intention to act only after the brain has readied itself to act and before the motor activity of the act itself. We can veto an action, but our intention to act is formulated in the brain before we become aware of it. In other words, we can't control what we feel but we can control how we act as a result of the feeling. The only way to change what we feel over time is to do the work of challenging the old schema that boxed up the feeling with other unusable thoughts, beliefs, and memories. In the meantime, it's important to use the body's conscious discipline to either select or inhibit the movement response to the feeling we are experiencing.

Lev Vygotsky and the zone of proximal development. Most books on human development will mention Lev Vygotsky, as well as materials about the history of education, but it might be best to just google him to read about it casually. He was one of the first people to talk about scaffolding, a support system in which a teacher creates conceptual structures that students can then climb on themselves toward understanding. This lies in contrast to just lecturing to students and their absorbing the information passively.

Chapter 2: The Anatomy of Bodyfulness

Stem cells. If you would like to learn more about stem cells, YouTube has some excellent short videos that explain and dramatize this amazing cell and its many processes. Just enter the term in their search engine.

Cell death. If you would like to learn more about cell death and its relationship to the death of an organism, see Sherwin B. Nuland, *How We Die* (New York: Vintage, 1995). It's an elegant and poetic book that helps us understand how the body navigates the death process from the cellular level onward.

Interbeing. The word *interbeing* was popularized by the Zen Buddhist master Thich Nhat Hanh. He writes extensively on this topic, but perhaps his most pointed references to this powerful term come in these books: *Being Peace* (Berkeley: Parallax Press, 2005); *Peace Is Every Step: The Path of Mindfulness in Everyday Life* (New York: Bantam, 1992); *The Miracle of Mindfulness* (Boston: Beacon Press, 1999).

Stress. Here is a wonderful, imminently readable book about stress, allostasis, and the effects of stress on the various systems of the body: Robert M. Sapolsky, *Why Zebra's Don't Get Ulcers*, 3rd ed. (New York: Henry Holt, 2004). Another researcher who advanced our understanding of stress was Hans Selye, an endocrinologist. He developed the concept of the general adaptation syndrome and coined the terms *stress*, *eustress*, and *distress*. Check him out if you want to learn more. His two most famous books: *The Stress of Life*, 2nd ed. (New York: McGraw-Hill, 1978) and *Stress Without Distress* (New York: Signet, 1975).

Polyvagal theory. Stephen W. Porges's polyvagal theory can be interesting and useful. His book *The Polyvagal Theory* is meant for people who already know anatomy and neuroscience. However, the pocket guide is touted as being more accessible: *The Pocket Guide to the Polyvagal Theory: The Transformative Power of Feeling Safe* (New York: W. W. Norton, 2017). Perhaps the best way to learn more about it is to simply look it up on Wikipedia or Google, as these explanations are more accessible.

Anatomical structures. Books that have good contemplative exercises that explore the anatomical divisions of the body and cultivate a subtler awareness of the interior of the body and what it's doing: Jeffrey Maitland, *Spacious Body: Explorations in Somatic Ontology* (Berkeley: North Atlantic Books, 1994); Richard Lowe and Stefan Laeng-Gilliatt, eds., *Reclaiming Vitality and Presence: Sensory Awareness as a Practice for Life* (Berkeley: North Atlantic Books, 2007); Andrea Olsen, *Body Stories: A Guide to Experiential Anatomy* (Lebanon, NH: University Press of New England, 2004); Deane Juhan, *Job's Body: A Handbook for Bodywork* (Barrytown, NY: Station Hill Press, 2003); Kathrin Stauffer, *Anatomy and Physiology for Psychotherapists: Connecting Body and Soul* (New York: W. W. Norton, 2010).

Automatic movements underlying voluntary movements. Some of the best writings about this principle come from Body-Mind Centering. Here are two of classic books: Linda Hartley, *Wisdom of the Body Moving: An Introduction to Body-Mind Centering* (Berkeley: North Atlantic Books, 1995); Bonnie Bainbridge Cohen, *Sensing, Feeling, and Action: The Experiential Anatomy of Body-Mind Centering* (Toronto: Contact Editions, 1994).

Chapter 3: Sensing

Sensory awareness. There are many fine somatic disciplines out there that we can use to work with sensory acuity. Some of the more well known: Focusing, developed by Eugene T. Gendlin; sensory awareness, developed by Charlotte Selver; the Rosen Method, developed by Marion Rosen; somatics, developed by Thomas Hanna.

Interoception and emotional intelligence. Research in this area was pioneered by Antonio Damasio and Joseph LeDoux and continued by Hugo Critchley. See Hugo D. Critchley, Stephan Wiens, Pia Rotshtein, Arne Öhman, and Raymond J. Dolan, "Neural Systems Supporting Interceptive Awareness," *Nature Neuroscience* 7, no. 2 (February 2004): 189–95. A more accessible article, one that pegs interoception to emotional intelligence, is Sandra Blakeslee and Matthew Blakeslee, "Where Mind and Body Meet," *Scientific American Mind* 18, no. 4 (August/September, 2007): 44–51, www.scientificamerican.com/article/where-mind-and-body-meet.

Body awareness and types of sensation. For a scholarly treatment of this topic, see the following for an excellent overview: Wolf E. Mehling, Virajini Gopisetty, Jennifer Daubenmier, Cynthia J. Price, Frederick M. Hecht, and Anita Stewart, "Body Awareness: Construct and Self-Report Measures," *PLoS ONE* 4, no. 5 (2009): e5614, doi:10.1371/journal.pone.0005614. Mehling states, for instance, that "a diffuse, emotion-based hypervigilance seems to be maladaptive, whereas 'concrete somatic monitoring' or 'sensory discrimination' of the precise details and present-moment characteristics in physical sensations appear to be adaptive."

Sensory richness. There are some lovely classic books that advocate for a rich sensory life. Three of the finest are: Morris Berman, *Coming to Our Senses: Body and Spirit in the Hidden History of the West* (New York: Bantam, 1989); David Abram, *The Spell of the Sensuous* (New York: Vintage, 1997); Diane Ackerman, *A Natural History of the Senses* (New York: Vintage, 1991).

Sensory processing disorders. These disorders are often discussed under the term *sensory integration.* The work of sensory integration often falls under the scope of practice of physical and occupational therapy, especially when treating children. Some classic and readable books on sensory integration: Carol Stock Kranowitz, *The Out-of-Sync Child Has Fun* (New York: TarcherPerigree, 2006); A. Jean Ayres, *Sensory Integration and Learning Disorders* (Los Angeles: Western Psychological Services, 1973).

Sensory processing. For a more scholarly approach to sensory awareness and processing, I would recommend Alan Fogel, *The Psychophysiology of Self-Awareness: Rediscovering the Lost Art of Body Sense* (New York: W.W. Norton, 2009) or *Body Sense: The Science and Practice of Embodied Self-Awareness* (New York: W.W. Norton, 2013).

Intuition. *The Journal of Consciousness Studies* publishes articles about intuition regularly. An author in that journal has written a dense but clear article that I recommend: Claire Petitmengin-Peugeot, "The Intuitive Experience," *Journal of Consciousness Studies* 6, no. 2–3 (1999): 43–77.

Chapter 4: Breathing

Physical and psychological benefits of breathing. Himmat K. Victoria and I have written two articles that attempt to provide a review of the theory and practice of therapeutic breathing: Christine Caldwell and Himmat K. Victoria, "Breathwork in Body Psychotherapy: Towards a More Unified Theory and Practice," *Body, Movement and Dance in Psychotherapy* 6, no. 2 (2011): 89–101; Himmat Kaur Victoria and Christine Caldwell, "Breathwork in Body Psychotherapy II: Clinical Applications," *Body, Movement, and Dance in Psychotherapy* 8, no. 4 (2013): 216–28.

Breath physiology. Robert Fried, with Joseph Grimaldi, *The Psychology and Physiology of Breathing: In Behavioral Medicine, Clinical Psychology, and Psychiatry* (New York: Plenum Press, 1993).

Breath anatomy. Blandine Calais-Germain, *Anatomy of Breathing* (Seattle: Eastland Press, 2006).

Breath and emotions. Susana Block, Madeleine Lemeignan, and Nancy Aquilera, "Specific Respiratory Patterns Distinguish among Human Basic Emotions," *International Journal of Psychophysiology* 11, no. 2 (August 1991): 141–54; Frans Boiten, "The Effects of Emotional Behaviour on Components of the Respiratory Cycle," *Biological Psychology* 49, no. 1–2 (September 1998): 29–51; Christopher

Gilbert, "Emotional Sources of Dysfunctional Breathing," *Journal of Bodywork and Movement Therapies* 2, no. 4 (October 1998): 224–330.

Breathing disorders. Leon Chaitow, Dinah Bradley, and Christopher Gilbert, *Multidisciplinary Approaches to Breathing Pattern Disorders* (London: Harcourt, 2002).

Good breathing practices. Donna Farhi, *The Breathing Book: Good Health and Vitality through Essential Breath Work* (New York: Henry Holt, 1996); Gay Hendricks, *Conscious Breathing: Breathwork for Health, Stress Release, and Personal Mastery* (New York: Bantam Books, 1995); Gay Hendricks and Kathlyn Hendricks, *Radiance: Breathwork, Movement & Body-Centered Psychotherapy* (Berkeley: Wingbow Press, 1991); Ilse Middendorf and Jureg Roffler, "The Breathing Self: The Experience of Breath as an Art to Healing Yourself," *International Journal of Yoga Therapy* 5, no. 1 (1994): 13–18.

Breath and spirituality. Peter Levine and Ian Macnaughton, "Breath and Consciousness: Reconsidering the Viability of Breathwork in Psychological and Spiritual Interventions in Human Development," in *Body, Breath, and Consciousness: A Somatics Anthology: A Collection of Articles on Family Systems, Self-Psychology, the Bodynamics Model of Somatic Developmental Psychology, Shock Trauma, and Breathwork,* ed. Ian Macnaughton (Berkeley: North Atlantic Books, 2004), 367–94.

Chapter 5: Moving

Falling and cognition in the elderly. The Oregon Brain Aging Study (Peter Wayne, Harvard Medical School) has found that there is a correlation between taking falls and cognitive impairment in the elderly, and the link between them is postural control. They also demonstrated that how you walk can diagnose cognitive decline. Improve postural control and you lessen falls and push back against cognitive decline. One suggestion was to challenge your balance while doing cognitive tasks.

Anatomical structures in movement. Blandine Calais-Germain, *Anatomy of Movement* (Seattle: Eastland Press, 2007).

Attention and movement. Dr. David Clark, at University of California, Berkeley, has studied attention deficit hyperactivity disorder (ADHD) and has also found a link between movement and cognition. ADHD, long considered to be a cognitive disorder, has been shown to have motor issues; in particular this study found that people with ADHD have trouble inhibiting nonessential actions when they move.

Animal and human play and play therapy. One of my favorite authors in this area is my friend Marc Bekoff. His publications in this area are too many to mention, but one of my favorites is Marc Bekoff and John Byers, eds., *Animal Play; Evolutionary, Comparative and Ecological Perspectives* (Cambridge, UK: Cambridge University Press, 1998). Other classics include Diane Ackerman, *Deep Play* (New York: Vintage, 2000); Robert M. Fagan, *Animal Play Behavior* (Oxford, UK: Oxford University Press, 1981); Charles Schaefer, ed., *Foundations of Play Therapy* (Hoboken, NJ: John-Wiley, 2003); Peter K. Smith, ed., *Play in Animals and Humans* (Hoboken, NJ: Blackwell, 1986).

Motor plans, reflexes, and fundamental movements. Body-Mind Centering, the work of Bonnie Bainbridge Cohen, has contributed greatly to our understanding of early and essential movements. Two of the classic books about it were listed in chapter 2's additional notes. Here is one other: Susan Aposhyan, *Natural Intelligence: Body-Mind Integration and Human Development* (Baltimore, MD: Williams & Wilkins, 1999).

Movement in trauma-based psychotherapies. Sensorimotor psychotherapy, a trauma-centered somatic psychotherapy method, comes highly recommended. Here are two great books about it: Pat Ogden, Kekuni Minton, and Clare Pain, *Trauma and the Body: A Sensorimotor Approach to Psychotherapy* (New York: W.W. Norton, 2006); Pat Ogden and Janina Fisher, *Sensorimotor Psychotherapy: Interventions for Trauma and Attachment* (New York: W.W. Norton, 2015). Also recommended: Peter Levine, *Waking the Tiger: Healing Trauma* (Berkeley: North Atlantic Books, 1997); Babette Rothschild, *The Body Remembers: The Psychophysiology of Trauma and Trauma Treatment* (New York: W.W. Norton, 2000).

Movement and early development. One of the best books in this area is this a thin volume: Ruella Frank and Frances La Barre, *The First Year and the Rest of Your Life: Movement, Development, and Psychotherapeutic Change* (New York: Routledge, 2011).

Nonverbal communication (NVC). For one of the early and enduring classics of NVC, see Nancy Henley, *Body Politics: Power, Sex, and Nonverbal Communication* (Upper Saddle River, NJ: Prentice Hall, 1986). Two more scholarly books in this area: Mark L. Knapp and Judith A. Hall, *Nonverbal Communication in Human Interaction* (Belmont, CA: Thomson Higher Education, 2006); John O'Neill, *The Communicative Body: Studies in Communicative Philosophy, Politics, and Sociology* (Evanston, IL: Northwestern University Press, 1989).

Posture and psychological states. Some areas of research focus more directly on body-centered practices or states as highly related to health and well-being—or the lack of it. For instance, it has been postulated that postural control problems may be a *core feature* of bipolar disorder, not just a random symptom. Researchers at Indiana University speculate that specific problems adapting to changing sensory input may lie at the core of this psychiatric disorder (Amanda Bolbecker et al., *Postural Control in Bipolar Disorder: Increased Sway Area and Decreased Dynamical Complexity*, https://doi.org/10.1371/journal.pone.0019824). This dovetails with various theories of schizophrenia that correlate it to sensory integration problems. Another good article is Richard E. Petty, Pablo Brinol, and Benjamin Wagner, "Body Posture Effects on Self-Evaluation: A Self-Validation Approach," *European Journal of Social Psychology* 39, no. 6 (2009): 1053–64.

Progressive relaxation. Most popular relaxation books will have a version of Edmund Jacobson's work in them. It may be useful to make a recording of your own voice guiding the progressive relaxation exercise. Jacobson's original work, which also tied in emotional processing as a function of body tone is *Biology of Emotions: New Understanding Derived from Biological Multidisciplinary Investigation; First Electrophysiological Measurements* (Springfield, IL: Charles C. Thomas, 1967).

Walking meditation. Many books on meditation will cover this wonderful practice. Thich Nhat Hanh, who is famous for his centralization of walking meditation, has several books on the subject, including this small book: *Walking Meditation: Peace is Every Step. It Turns the Endless Path to Joy* (Boulder, CO: Sounds True, 2006).

Chapter 6: Relating

Early caregiver interactions. M. Bullowa, "When Infant and Adult Communicate How Do They Synchronize Their Behaviors?" in *Organization of Behavior in Face-to-Face Interaction,* ed. Adam Kendon, Richard M. Harris, and Mary Key (Chicago: Aldine Publishing Company, 1975).

Parents as "external psychobiological regulators." Allan N. Schore, *Affect Regulation and the Origin of the Self: The Neurobiology of Emotional Development* (Mahwah, NJ: Lawrence Erlbaum Associates, 1994).

Play behavior. See my chapter on adult group play therapy to give you some idea of the stages of contemplative play: Christine Caldwell, "Adult Group Play Therapy," in *Play Therapy with Adults,* ed. Charles E. Schaefer (Hoboken, NJ: John Wiley and Sons, 2003), 301–16.

Enduring physical tendencies. A good discussion of this topic can be found in Pat Ogden, Kekuni Minton, and Clare Pain, *Trauma and the Body: A Sensorimotor Approach to Psychotherapy* (New York: W.W. Norton, 2006).

Body boundaries, borders, and defenses. The idea of body boundaries being related to our sense of our borders and limits got started with body image researchers in the 1950s and '60s. Check out Fisher and Cleveland for that. More recently, this idea was taken up by various body psychotherapists, most notably Stanley Keleman and Jack Lee Rosenberg & Marjorie Rand.

Touch. Dr. Tiffany Fields has been the go-to researcher on touch. She has spent much of her career at the University of Florida, researching the effects of touch deprivation on infants, particularly hospitalized infants.

Body attunement and coregulation. These ideas have mostly been studied by psychotherapists and developmental psychologists. Allan N. Schore, cited just above in the "parents as external psychobiological regulators" section, holds perhaps the most extensive referencing of the research literature on coregulation with infants and children. For adults, one of the best books has been written by psychotherapist David J. Wallin, *Attachment in Psychotherapy* (New York: Guilford Press, 2007).

Chapter 7: Body Identity, Body Authority, and Bodyful Stories

Narrative identity. If you are feeling very scholarly, here are three great articles on narrative identity: Dan P. McAdams, Ruthellen Josselson, and Amia Lieblich, eds., *Identity and Story: Creating Self in Narrative* (Washington, DC: American Psychological Association, 2006); Hubert J. M. Hermans, "The Dialogical Self: Toward a Theory of Personal and Cultural Positioning," *Culture and Psychology* 7, no. 3 (2001): 243–81; Dan P. McAdams, *The Redemptive Self* (New York: Oxford University Press, 2013).

Body memory. A more thorough article on this topic can be found in Christine Caldwell, "Sensation, Movement, and Emotion: Explicit Procedures for Implicit Memories," in *Body Memory, Metaphor and Movement*, eds. Sabine C. Koch, Thomas Fuchs, Michela Summa, M., and Cornelia Muller (Amsterdam: John Benjamins, 2012), 255–66.

Body authority. While I have written elsewhere on this topic, I received my inspiration for this idea from the work of anthropologist Brigitte Jordon, who researched childbirth in different cultures and how women in technologically advanced societies give up the authoritative knowledge of their bodies when they enter hospital maternity wards. One of the best books on the topic is Robbie E. Davis-Floyd and Carolyn F. Sargent, eds., *Childbirth and Authoritative Knowledge: Cross-Cultural Perspectives* (Berkeley: University of California Press, 1997).

Body identity and body narratives. Christine Caldwell, "Body Identity Development: Definitions and Discussions," *Body, Movement, and Dance in Psychotherapy* 11, no. 4 (2016): 220–34.

Authoritative knowledge of the body—nonverbal communication. A classic text: Nancy Henley, *Body Politics: Power, Sex, and Nonverbal Communication* (Upper Saddle River, NJ: Prentice Hall, 1986).

Morality. Though a bit older, this book discusses the ways in which our sociality and our "animal natures" can urge us toward a moral life: Robert Wright, *The Moral Animal: Why We Are the Way We Are: The New Science of Evolutionary Psychology* (New York: Vintage Books, 1994).

Movement inquiry. While I have been teaching this concept for many years, I haven't written on it. In many ways, the movement inquiry practice owes its shape and form to a type of dance therapy called Authentic Movement. This self-directed way of exploring emergent movement impulses was developed by Mary Starks Whitehouse. A good book on the topic: Patrizia Pallaro, ed., *Authentic Movement: A Collection of Essays by Mary Starks Whitehouse, Janet Adler and Joan Chodorow* (Philadelphia: Jessica Kingsley Publishers, 1999).

Chapter 8: Bodylessness and the Reclamation of Bodily Authority

How bodylessness gets started. My first book, *Getting Our Bodies Back*, goes into greater detail about addictive experiences in the body: how they develop, how they are maintained, and how we can recover from them. The book is premised on an early notion of bodylessness as the core feature of addictive experiences.

Christine Caldwell, *Getting Our Bodies Back* (Boston: Shambhala Publications, 1996).

Contemplative body practices as an anti-oppression strategy. An academic article by Deborah Orr might be useful as a means to understand ways in which body oppression influences how we learn and our educational systems. She advocates for body-based practices such as yoga and tai chi as ways to access knowledge differently and as means to resist the hegemony of mentalizing. Deborah Orr, "The Uses of Mindfulness in Anti-Oppressive Pedagogies: Philosophy and Praxis," *Canadian Journal of Education* 27, no. 4 (2002): 477–90.

Darwin's threat to human exceptionalism. This idea can be widely accessed, but a classic book that can get you started is Daniel C. Dennett, *Darwin's Dangerous Idea: Evolution and the Meanings of Life* (New York: Simon & Schuster, 1995).

The oppressed and marginalized body. Lucy Bennett Leighton and I coedited *Oppression and the Body: Roots, Resistance, and Resolutions* (Berkeley: North Atlantic Books, 2018). The book includes various authors who examine how we oppress bodies in general, how we oppress specific bodies, and what we can do to reclaim our embodied natures as a form of resistance.

Chapter 9: When Being Here Takes You There

Mindfulness and acceptance-based therapies. For a great read on these psychotherapies, I recommend Christopher K. Germer, Ronald D. Siegel, and Paul R. Fulton, eds., *Mindfulness & Psychotherapy* (New York: Guilford Press, 2005).

Exercise and emotional health. Moderate exercise is good for all sorts of psychiatric disorders, such as anxiety, depression, alcohol dependence, chronic pain, even schizophrenia. It compares favorably to individual and group psychotherapy, and cognitive therapy. See Gregg A. Tkachuk and Garry L. Martin, "Exercise Therapy for Patients with Psychiatric Disorders: Research and Clinical Implications," *Professional Psychology: Research and Practice* 30, no. 3 (1999): 275–82. Multiple studies show a strong relationship between exercise or dance and a lessening of depression or anxiety and an improvement in certain types of memory (Leste & Rust, 1984; Martinsen & Solberg, 1989; Nakamura et al., 2007). Combining dance/movement therapy and yoga has been shown to increase stress management and communication skills, as well as ameliorate prosocial behaviors (Barton, 2011).

Body awareness and emotional intelligence. Another study found that body awareness training assisted emotional processing (Sze et al., 2010), and a qualitative study found that developing a heightened sense of bodily movement "engenders an interconnected, bodily grounded sense of cultural identity" (Caroline Potter, "Sense of Motion, Senses of Self: Becoming a Dancer," 2008, www.tandfonline.com/doi/abs/10.1080/00141840802563915).

Pleasure. Warren, Brown and Ryan (2003 and 2007) found that people with more mindfulness felt pleasure more frequently and intensely, felt bad less often and less intensely, and felt more autonomous about their daily activities.

Martial arts and attention. Other researchers who included martial arts in their construct of mindfulness as they studied troubled adolescents found improvements in ADHD symptoms and relationships to parents, as well as decreased anxiety. See Jillian Haydicky, Judith Weiner, Paul Bdali, Karen Miligan, and Joseph M. Ducharme, "Evaluation of a Mindfulness-Based Intervention for Adolescents with Learning Disabilities and Co-Occurring ADHD and Anxiety," *Mindfulness* 3, no. 2 (June 2012): 151–64.

Having an "upper limit" setting on pleasure. The concept of an upper limits problem was popularized by Gay and Kathlyn Hendricks, in their classic book *Conscious Loving: The Journey to Commitment* (New York: Bantam, 1990).

Flow states/creative states. The person who coined the term *flow* is Mihaly Csikszentmihalyi, from the University of Chicago. Best to start with his work: *Flow: The Psychology of Optimal Experience* (New York: Harper, 2008).

Chapter 10. The Enlightened Body

Bodyfulness research. Meta-analyses of mind-body studies reveal a widening of beneficial effects, including a decrease in migraine headaches, fibromyalgia, multiple sclerosis, epilepsy, stroke, and Parkinson's disease. Practices included in the definition of mind-body therapy were meditation, relaxation, conscious breathing, yoga, tai chi, qigong, hypnosis, and biofeedback (Wahbeh et al., 2008). Obviously this is a very wide and inclusive net, spanning both top-down and bottom-up techniques, but it again points to the possible usefulness of present-centered, experiential practices that involve the body (via sensory awareness and movement) and involves a capacity to pay high-quality attention.

Mind-body practices and physical health. Another meta-analysis of mind-body medicine treatments, which included relaxation, cognitive behavioral therapies, meditation, imagery, biofeedback, and hypnosis, found considerable evidence of efficacy in the areas of reducing coronary heart disease, headaches, insomnia, incontinence, chronic lower back pain, disease and treatment-related symptoms of cancer, and improved postsurgical outcomes (Astin et al., 2003).

Recollective awareness meditation. This is a meditation form developed by Jason Siff. It consists of three components: an intent to meditate, a purposeful posture, and some place to come back to in order to ground you when you wander. Siff feels that meditation is about where you place your attention. Thoughts and emotions begin to settle down naturally as awareness of the body and the breath move into the foreground. He asks us to question the labels we put on thoughts, such as anger or depression. What is the experience without the label? He encourages us to not remain detached, to not separate from thoughts or try to stop them. Instead, he encourages us to get involved. This method shares many features with bodyfulness as we understand it (Siff, 2014).

Sweat your prayers. This lovely statement formed the title of a 1998 book by Gabrielle Roth, a movement and theater artist who developed a form of movement-based personal and spiritual development called 5Rhythms. This practice constitutes a great example of combining one's joy in moving with discernment and practice, in the service of waking up the body in motion (Gabrielle Roth, *Sweat Your Prayers: The Five Rhythms of the Soul—Movement as Spiritual Practice*, New York: Toucher/Putnam, 1997).

Bibliography

Aposhyan, Susan. *Natural Intelligence: Body-Mind Integration and Human Development.* Baltimore, MD: Williams & Wilkins, 1999.

Astin, J., S. Shapiro, D. Eisenberg, and K. Forys. "Mind-Body Medicine: State of Science, Implications for Practice." *Journal of the American Board of Family Medicine* 16, no. 2 (March 1, 2003): 131–47.

Ayres, A. Jean. *Sensory Integration and Learning Disorders.* Los Angeles: Western Psychological Services, 1973.

Baer, Ruth A., James Carmody, and Matthew Hunsinger. "Weekly Change in Mindfulness and Perceived Stress in a Mindfulness-Based Stress Reduction Program." *Journal of Clinical Psychology* 68, no. 7 (July 2012): 755–65. doi:10.1002/jclp.21865.

Barton, Emma J. "Movement and Mindfulness: A Formative Evaluation of a Dance/Movement and Yoga Therapy Program with Participants Experiencing Severe Mental Illness." *American Journal of Dance Therapy* 33, no. 2 (December 2011): 157–81.

Berman, Morris. *Coming to Our Senses: Body and Spirit in the Hidden History of the West.* New York: Bantam, 1989.

Bollas, Christopher. *The Shadow of the Object: Psychoanalysis of the Unthought Known.* New York: Columbia University Press, 1987.

Boorstein, Sylvia. *Don't Just Do Something, Sit There: A Mindfulness Retreat with Sylvia Boorstein*. San Francisco: HarperCollins, 1996.

Brown, Kirk Warren, and Richard M. Ryan. "The Benefits of Being Present: Mindfulness and Its Role in Psychological Wellbeing." *Journal of Personality and Social Psychology* 84, no. 4 (2003): 822–48.

Brown, Kirk Warren, Richard M. Ryan, and J. David Creswell. "Mindfulness: Theoretical Foundations and Evidence for Its Salutary Effects." *Psychological Inquiry* 18, no. 4 (2007): 211–37.

Burg, Jan M., Oliver T. Wolf, and Johannes Michalak. "Mindfulness as Self-Regulated Attention: Associations with Heart Rate Variability." *Swiss Journal of Psychology* 71, no. 3 (2012): 135–39.

Butler, Judith. *Bodies That Matter: On the Discursive Limits of "Sex."* New York: Routledge, 1993.

Caldwell, Christine. "Adult Group Play Therapy." In *Play Therapy with Adults*, edited by Charles E. Schaefer, 301–16. Hoboken, NJ: John Wiley and Sons, 2003.

Caldwell, Christine. "Body Identity Development: Definitions and Discussions." *Body, Movement, and Dance in Psychotherapy* 11, no. 4 (2016): 220–34. doi: 10.1080/17432979.2016.1145141.

Caldwell, Christine, ed. "Body Identity Development: Who We Are and Who We Become." *Oppression and the Body*, edited by Christine Caldwell and Lucia Bennett Leighton. Berkeley, CA: North Atlantic Books, 2018: 31–50.

Caldwell, Christine. "Conscious Movement Sequencing: The Core of the Dance Movement Psychotherapy Experience." In *Essentials of Dance Movement Psychotherapy: International Perspectives on Theory, Research, and Practice*, edited by Helen Payne, 51–64. London: Routledge, 2017.

Caldwell, Christine. "Diversity Issues in Movement Observation and Assessment." *American Journal of Dance Therapy* 35, no. 2 (2013): 183–200. doi:10.1007/s10465-013-9159-9.

Caldwell, Christine. *Getting Our Bodies Back.* Boston: Shambhala Publications, 1996.

Caldwell, Christine. "Mindfulness and Bodyfulness: A New Paradigm." *Journal of Contemplative Inquiry* 1, no. 1 (2014): 77–96.

Caldwell, Christine. "Sensation, Movement, and Emotion: Explicit Procedures for Implicit Memories." In *Body Memory, Metaphor and Movement*, edited by Sabine C. Koch, Thomas Fuchs, Michela Summa, and Cornelia Muller, 255–66. Amsterdam: John Benjamins, 2012.

Caldwell, Christine, and Himmat K. Victoria. "Breathwork in Body Psychotherapy: Towards a More Unified Theory and Practice." *Body, Movement and Dance in Psychotherapy* 6, no. 2 (2011): 89–101.

Chiesa, Alberto, Paolo Brambila, and Alessandro Seretti. "Functional Neural Correlates of Mindfulness Meditations in Comparison with Psychotherapy, Pharmacotherapy and Placebo Effect. Is There a Link?" *Acta Neuropsychiatrica* 22, no. 3 (2010): 104–17.

Critchley, Hugo D., Stephan Wiens, Pia Rotshtein, Arne Öhman, and Raymond J. Dolan. "Neural Systems Supporting Interceptive Awareness." *Nature Neuroscience* 7, no. 2 (February 2004): 189–95.

Csikszentmihaly, Mihaly. *Flow: The Psychology of Optimal Experience.* New York: Harper, 2008.

Damasio, Antonio. *Self Comes to Mind: Constructing the Conscious Brain.* New York: Vintage Books, 2012.

Davidson, Richard J., Jon Kabat-Zinn, Jessica R. Schumacher, Melissa Rosen-kranz, Daniel Muller, Saki Santorelli, Ferris Urbanowski, Anne Harrington, Katherine Bonus, and John F. Sheridan. "Alterations in Brain and Immune Function Produced by Mindfulness Meditation." *Psychosomatic Medicine* 65, no. 4 (2003): 564–70.

Davis, Daphne M., and Jeffrey A. Hayes. "What Are the Benefits of Mindfulness? A Practice Review of Psychotherapy-Related Research." *Psychotherapy* 48, no. 2 (2011): 198–208.

Davis-Floyd, Robbie E., and Carolyn F. *Childbirth and Authoritative Knowledge: Cross-Cultural Perspectives.* Berkeley: University of California Press, 1997.

Eddy, Martha. *Mindful Movement: The Evolution of the Somatic Arts and Conscious Action.* Chicago: University of Chicago Press, 2016.

Erikson, Erik H. *Childhood and Society.* 2nd ed. New York: Norton, 1963.

Farb, Norman A. S., Adam K. Anderson, Helen Mayberg, Jim Bean, Deborah McKeon, and Zindel V. Segal. "Minding One's Emotions: Mindfulness Training Alters the Neural Expression of Sadness." *Emotion* 10, no. 1 (February 2010): 25–33.

Field, Tiffany. *Touch.* Cambridge, MA: MIT Press, 2001.

Fogel, Alan. *The Psychophysiology of Self-Awareness: Rediscovering the Lost Art of Body Sense.* New York: W.W. Norton, 2009.

Fosha, Diana. *The Transforming Power of Affect: A Model for Accelerated Change.* New York: Basic Books, 2000.

Frank, Ruella, and Frances La Barre. *The First Year and the Rest of Your Life: Movement, Development, and Psychotherapeutic Change.* New York: Routledge, 2011.

Gallagher, Shaun. (2014). "Phenomenology and Embodied Cognition." In *The Routledge Handbook of Embodied Cognition*, edited by Lawrence Shapiro, 9–18. London: Routledge, 2014.

Gazzaniga, Michael S. "Cerebral Specialization and Interhemispheric Communication." *Brain* 123, no. 7 (July 2000): 1293–1326.

Germer, Christopher K., Ronald D. Siegel, and Paul R. Fulton, eds. *Mindfulness & Psychotherapy*. New York: Guilford Press, 2005.

Goldin, Philippe R., and James J. Gross. "Effects of Mindfulness-Based Stress Reduction (MBSR) on Emotion Regulation in Social Anxiety Disorder." *Emotion* 10, no. 1 (February 2010): 83–91.

Green, Sheryl M., and Peter J. Bieling. "Expanding the Scope of Mindfulness-Based Cognitive Therapy: Evidence for Effectiveness in a Heterogeneous Psychiatric Sample." *Cognitive and Behavioral Practice* 19, no. 1 (2012): 174–80. doi:10.1016/j.cbpra.2011.02.006.

Grepmair, Ludwig, Ferdinand Meitterlehner, Thomas Loew, Egon Bachler, Wolfhardt Rother, and Marius Nickel. "Promoting Mindfulness in Psychotherapists in Training Influences the Treatment Results of Their Patients: A Randomized, Double-Blind, Controlled Study." *Psychotherapy and Psychosomatics* 76, no. 6 (2007): 332–38. doi:10.1159/000107560.

Hanna, Thomas. *The Body of Life*. New York: Alfred A. Knopf, 1979.

Hanna, Thomas. *Somatics: Reawakening the Mind's Control of Movement, Flexibility, and Health*. New York: Addison-Wesley Company, 1988.

Hannaford, Carla. *Smart Moves: Why Learning Is Not All in Your Head*. Arlington, VA: Great Ocean Publishers, 2005.

Haydicky, Jillian, Judith Weiner, Paul Bdali, Karen Miligan, and Joseph M. Ducharme. "Evaluation of a Mindfulness-Based Intervention for Adolescents with Learning Disabilities and Co-Occurring ADHD and Anxiety." *Mindfulness* 3, no. 2 (June 2012): 151–64.

Hermans, Hubert J. M. "The Dialogical Self: Toward a Theory of Personal and Cultural Positioning." *Culture and Psychology* 7, no. 3 (2001): 243–81.

Jackson, Linda. "Physical Attractiveness: A Sociocultural Perspective." In *Body Image: A Handbook of Theory, Research, and Clinical Practice*, edited by Thomas F. Cash and Thomas Pruzinsky, 13–2. New York: Guilford Press, 2002.

Jha, Amishi P., Elizabeth A. Stanley, Anastasia Kiyonaga, Ling Wong, and Lis Gelfand. "Examining the Protective Effects of Mindfulness Training on Working Memory Capacity and Affective Experience." *Emotion* 10, no. 1 (February 2010): 54–64.

Johnson, Don Hanlon. *Body, Spirit and Democracy.* Berkeley: North Atlantic Books, 1994.

Kabat-Zinn, Jon. *Full Catastrophe Living: Using the Wisdom of Your Body and Mind to Face Stress, Pain, and Illness.* New York: Delta, 1991.

Kabat-Zinn, Jon. "Mindfulness-Based Interventions in Context: Past, Present, and Future." *Clinical Psychology Science and Practice* 10, no. 2 (June 2003): 144–56.

Kabat-Zinn, Jon, Leslie Lipworth, and Robert Burney. "The Clinical Use of Mindfulness Meditation for the Self-Regulation of Chronic Pain." *Journal of Behavioral Medicine* 8, no. 2 (June 1985): 163–90.

Keng, Shian-Ling, Moria J. Smoski, and Clive Robins. "Effects of Mindfulness on Psychological Health: A Review of Empirical Studies." *Clinical Psychology Review* 31, no. 6 (August 2011): 1041–56. doi:10.1016/j.cpr.2011.04.006.

Knapp, Mark L., and Judith A. Hall. *Nonverbal Communication in Human Interaction*. Belmont, CA: Thomson Higher Education, 2006.

Kopp, Sheldon. *Back to One: A Practical Guide for Psychotherapists*. Palo Alto, CA: Science and Behavior Books, 1977.

LeDoux, Joseph. *The Emotional Brain: The Mysterious Underpinnings of Emotional Life*. New York: Simon & Schuster, 1996.

Lefevre, Carole. "Posture, Muscular Tone and Visual Attention in 5-Month-Old Infants." *Infant and Child Development* 11, no. 4 (December 2002): 335–46.

Leste Andre, and John Rust. "Effects of Dance on Anxiety." *Perceptual and Motor Skills* 58, no. 3 (June 1984): 767–72.

Libet, Benjamin, "Do We Have Free Will?" *Journal of Consciousness Studies* 6, no. 8–9 (August 1, 1999): 47–57.

Lutz, Antoine, Lawrence L. Greischar, Nancy B. Rawlings, Matthieu Ricard, and Richard J. Davidson. "Long-Term Meditators Self-Induce High-Amplitude Gamma Synchrony during Mental Practice." *Proceedings of the National Academy of Sciences* 101, no. 46 (November 16, 2004): 16369–73.

Martinsen, Egil W., Asle Hoffart, and Yvind Solberg. "Aerobic and Non-Aerobic Forms of Exercise in the Treatment of Anxiety Disorders." *Stress Medicine* 5, no. 2 (April 1989): 115–20. doi:10.1002/smi.2460050209.

McAdams, Dan P., Ruthellen Josselson, and Amia Lieblich, eds. *Identity and Story: Creating Self in Narrative*. Washington, DC: American Psychological Association, 2006.

Mehling, Wolf E., Virajini Gopisetty, Jennifer Daubenmier, Cynthia J. Price, Frederick M. Hecht, and Anita Stewart. "Body Awareness: Construct and Self-Report Measures." *PLoS ONE* 4, no. 5 (2009): e5614. doi:10.1371/journal.pone.0005614.

Michalak, Johannes, Nikolaus Troje, and Thomas Heidenreich. "The Effects of Mindfulness-Based Cognitive Therapy on Depressive Gait Patterns." *Journal of Cognitive and Behavioral Psychotherapies* 11, no. 1 (March 2011): 13–27.

Nakamura, Toru, Hideaki Soya, Custer C. Deocaris, Akiyo Kimpara, Miho Iimura, Takahiko Fujikawa, Hyukki Chang, Bruce S. McEwen, and Takeshi Nishijima. "BDNF Induction with Mild Exercise in the Rat Hippocampus." *Biochemical Biophysical Research Community* 358, no. 4 (July 13, 2007): 961–67.

Ogden, Pat, Kekuni Minton, and Clare Pain. *Trauma and the Body: A Sensorimotor Approach to Psychotherapy.* New York: W.W. Norton, 2006.

Oliver, Mary. *New and Selected Poems.* Boston: Beacon Press, 1992.

Orr, Deborah. "The Uses of Mindfulness in Anti-Oppressive Pedagogies: Philosophy and Praxis." *Canadian Journal of Education* 27, no. 4 (2002): 477–90.

Pallaro, Patrizia, ed. *Authentic Movement: A Collection of Essays by Mary Starks Whitehouse, Janet Adler and Joan Chodorow.* Philadelphia: Jessica Kingsley Publishers, 1999.

Pert, Candace. *The Molecules of Emotion: The Science Behind Mind-Body Medicine.* New York: Touchstone, 1997.

Porges, Stephen W. "The Polyvagal Theory: Phylogenetic Substrates of a Social Nervous System." *International Journal of Psychophysiology* 42, no. 2 (October 2001): 123–46.

Ramel, Wiveka, Philippe R. Goldin, Paula E. Carmona, and John R. McQuaid. "The Effects of Mindfulness Meditation on Cognitive Processes and Affect in Patients with Past Depression." *Cognitive Therapy and Research* 28, no. 4 (August 2004): 433–55.

Robbins, Michael W. "Scientists See Yet Another Reason to Go to the Gym." *Discover Magazine* (January 2004). http://discovermagazine.com/2004/jan/neuroscience#.UtLssJ5dWSo.

Rosenberg, Jack Lee, and Marjorie Rand. *Body, Self, and Soul: Sustaining Integration*. Atlanta, GA: Humanics Trade Group, 1985.

Schore, Allan N. *Affect Regulation and the Origin of the Self: The Neurobiology of Emotional Development*. Mahwah, NJ: Lawrence Erlbaum Associates, 1994.

Sherrell, Carla. "The Oppression of Black Bodies: The Demand to Simulate White Bodies and White Embodiment." *Oppression and the Body: Roots, Resistances, and Resolutions*, edited by Christine Caldwell and Lucia Bennett Leighton. Berkeley, CA: North Atlantic Press, 2018: 141–56.

Shusterman, Richard. *Body Consciousness: A Philosophy of Mindfulness and Somaesthetics*. New York: Cambridge University Press, 2008.

Siegel, Daniel J. *The Mindful Brain: Reflection and Attunement in the Cultivation of Well-Being*. New York: W.W. Norton, 2007.

Siff, Jason. *Thoughts Are Not the Enemy: An Innovative Approach to Meditation*. Boulder, CO: Shambhala Publications, 2014.

Silow, T. Personal communication, USABP Conference, Boulder, CO, August 12, 2012.

Smalley, Susan, L., Sandra K. Loo, T. Sigi Halle, Anshu Shrestha, James McGough, Lisa Flook, and Steven Reise. "Mindfulness and Attention Deficit Hyperactivity Disorder." *Journal of Clinical Psychology* 65, no. 10 (October 2009): 1087–98.

Stern, Daniel N. *The Present Moment in Psychotherapy and Everyday Life*. New York: W.W. Norton, 2004.

Sugamura, G., H. Takase, Y. Haruki, and F. Koshikawa. "Bodyfulness and Posture: It's Concept and Some Empirical Support." Poster presentation at the 65th Convention of the International Council of Psychologists, San Diego, CA, December 2007.

Sugamura, G., Y. Haruki, and F. Koshikawa. "Mindfulness and Bodyfulness in the Practices of Meditation: A Comparison of Western and Eastern Theories of Mind-Body." Poster presentation at the First Convention of the Asian Psychological Association, Bali, Indonesia, June 2006.

Sze, Jocelyn A., Anett Gyurak, Joyce W. Yuan, and Robert W. Levenson. "Coherence between Emotional Experience and Physiology: Does Body Awareness Training Have an Impact?" *Emotion* 10, no. 6 (December 2010): 803–14.

Tiggemann, Marika. "Media Influences on Body Image Development." In *Body Image: A Handbook of Theory, Research, and Clinical Practice*, edited by Thomas F. Cash and Thomas Pruzinsky, 91–98. New York: Guilford Press, 2002.

van der Oord, Saskia, Susan M. Bögels, and Dorreke Peijnenburg. "The Effectiveness of Mindfulness Training for Children with ADHD and Mindful Parenting for Their Parents." *Journal of Child and Family Studies* 21, no. 1 (February 2012): 139–47. doi: 10.1007/s10826-011-9457-0.

Victoria, H. Kaur, and Christine Caldwell. "Breathwork in Body Psychotherapy: Clinical Applications." *Body, Movement and Dance in Psychotherapy* 8, no. 4 (2013): 216–28.

Wahbeh, Helané, Elsas Siegward-M, and Barry S. Oken. "Mind-Body Interventions." *Neurology* 70, no. 24 (June 2008): 2321–28.

Wallace, B. Alan. *The Attention Revolution: Unlocking the Power of the Focused Mind.* Boston: Wisdom Publications, 2006.

Wallin, David J. *Attachment in Psychotherapy.* New York: Guilford Press, 2007.

Weisbuch, Max, and Kristin Pauker. "The Nonverbal Transmission of Intergroup Bias: A Model of Bias Contagion with Implications for Social Policy." *Social Issues and Policy Review* 5, no. 1 (December 2011): 257–91.

Welwood, John. *Toward a Psychology of Awakening: Buddhism, Psychotherapy, and the Path of Personal and Spiritual Transformation.* Boston: Shambhala Publications, 2000.

Wilkinson, Margaret. *Changing Minds in Therapy: Emotion, Attachment, Trauma, and Neurobiology.* New York: W.W. Norton, 2010.

Williams, J., "Mindfulness and Psychological Process." *Emotion* 10, no. 1 (February 2010): 1–7. doi:10.1037/a0018360.

Wittgenstein, Ludwig. *Philosophical Investigations.* Oxford, UK: Basil Blackwell, 1968.

Woollacott, Marjorie, and Anne Shumway-Cook. "Attention and the Control of Posture and Gait: A Review of an Emerging Area of Research." *Gait and Posture* 16, no. 1 (August 2002): 1–14.

Yuasa, Yasuo. *The Body: Toward an Eastern Mind-Body Theory.* New York: SUNY Press, 1987.

Index